AF439971

Muscle Building Shortcut

NO Heavy Weights or Long Gym Hours

Beginners, Injured, Elderly, and Athletes

by

Dr. Janeil Stehr, PT, DPT, CSCS

Although the author and publisher have made every effort to ensure that the information in this book was correct at press time, the author and publisher do not assume and hereby disclaim any liability to any party for any loss, damage, or disruption caused by errors or omissions, whether such errors or omissions result from negligence, accident, or any other cause.

This publication is designed to provide accurate and authoritative information with regard to the subject matter covered. It is sold with the understanding that the publisher is not engaged in rendering professional services. If legal advice or other expert assistance is required, the services of a competent professional should be sought. This work is published with the understanding that the author and publisher are providing information but are not attempting to render medical or other professional services. The information contained within this book is strictly for educational and entertainment purposes. Therefore, if you wish to apply ideas contained in this book, you are taking full responsibility for your actions. It is the responsibility of the reader to consult a licensed professional before attempting any of the techniques outlined in this book. Using the concepts and procedures presented may be beyond some people's physical abilities and could result in injury. Those engaging in the proposed activities should do so within safe and appropriate limits and seek medical advice if they have any concerns about their personal health.

The fact that an organization or website is referred to in this work as a citation and/or a potential source of further information does not mean that the author or the publisher endorses the information the organization or website may provide or recommendations it may make. This book cites various sources in line with academic standards. These sources are for informational purposes and to attribute ideas and concepts to their originating authors, as is customary in scholarly writing.

Please remember that internet websites listed in this work may have changed or removed between when this work was written and when it is read. By reading this book, you agree that you have read and understand the aforementioned disclaimer.

Table of Contents

Introduction

Welcome to a realm of fitness that defies the traditional norms of muscle building and endurance training. You are about to uncover a method that can help anybody—from the hardcore bodybuilder to the senior looking to maintain muscle mass—achieve significant fitness results without spending countless hours in the gym or lifting heavy weights. This cutting-edge method is called blood occlusion training (BOT), a scientifically proven technique that can trick the body into responding as if

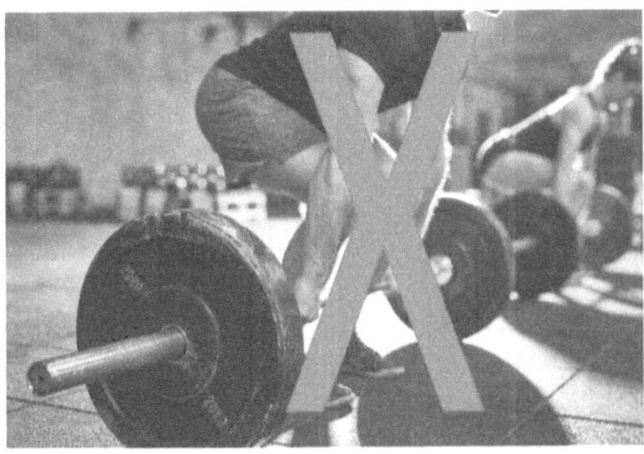

it is undergoing heavy lifting when it is NOT!

The concept of BOT is intriguing, yet it might sound counterintuitive or even daunting at first. After all, "blood occlusion" appears a bit extreme, implying a process far removed from the healthy, circulation-friendly exercises we are accustomed to. But I assure you, this method is grounded in solid science; it is a carefully calibrated approach that involves the strategic application of pressure to the body's extremities during low-intensity workouts which elicits a surge of muscle building responses in the body.

Perhaps you are an athlete seeking to gain a competitive edge, a military member looking to maintain peak physical condition, an amputee or someone recovering from an injury. Maybe you are an older adult aiming to preserve strength and muscle tissue, or simply someone who is hit a plateau in their regular routine. Regardless of your starting point, this Introduction is your gateway to understanding how BOT stands out in the crowd of fitness strategies.

Now, let us clarify what BOT is not. It is not a shortcut to avoid the hard work that fitness requires. Nor is it magic. BOT necessitates precision, understanding, and a respect for the boundaries of one's own body. It is a different path to the same summit of physical achievement. What makes it special is its efficiency and accessibility; it is a way to achieve more with less strain.

The science behind BOT revolves around the concept of restricting venous blood flow out of the muscle while still permitting arterial blood flow into the muscle (Takarada et al., 2000). This temporary blood flow restriction, achieved using special bands or cuffs, leads to blood pooling within the muscle. This condition challenges the muscle, even under low-intensity exercise, and encourages growth similar to high-intensity resistance training.

For those who are intimidated by heavy weights or are unable to use them due to medical conditions or 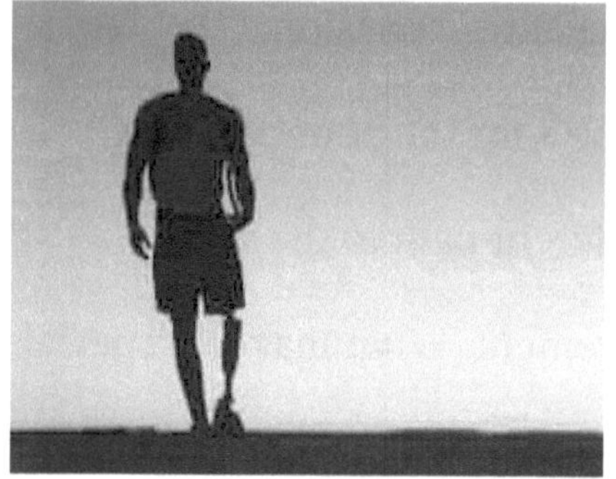 injuries, BOT represents a beacon of hope. It can be utilized to maintain or increase muscle size and strength when lifting heavy weights is not an option. This makes it not only an incredibly versatile tool in the fitness arsenal, but also for the injured and elderly.

Implementation of BOT is not a one-size-fits-all solution. It must be tailored to each individual, and this book will guide you through the necessary steps to safely and effectively adopt this method. We will dive into the specific protocols suitable for varied groups—yes, including protocols for athletes, the injured, and military personnel, which will be discussed in-depth in the coming chapters.

Moreover, for special populations such as the elderly, BOT can be a game-changer. With age, muscle atrophy is a common concern, and maintaining muscle function is key to preserving autonomy. BOT offers a means to stimulate muscle growth without the risks associated with heavy lifting (Karabulut et al., 2010).

While the focus of this book is largely on muscle development and endurance, it is also critical to understand the broader ecosystem of fitness in which BOT operates. Nutrition and recovery are just as essential to this method as they are to any other training regimen. After all, muscles need the right fuel to grow and the appropriate rest to repair and strengthen.

Now you might wonder if BOT is really as effective as traditional resistance training methods. The answer is supported by numerous scientific studies demonstrating significant increases in muscle size and strength with BOT—results similar to those achieved with high-intensity resistance training (Loenneke et al., 2012).

But every silver lining has a cloud; and it is important to address potential drawbacks and how to manage them. The safety measures and best practices highlighted later in this book will provide a framework ensuring you reap the benefits of BOT without incurring unnecessary risk.

This Introduction is just the surface skim of a deep and fascinating pool of knowledge surrounding blood occlusion training. As the pages unfold, so too will the nuance and potential of this remarkable method. Let us then embark on a journey that promises to expand your understanding and application of this innovative avenue to muscular development.

The road to achieving significant fitness milestones need not always be paved with heavy weight and sweat. BOT offers a different route—a scientific, smart, and strategic path that is inclusive and adaptable to a variety of needs and ambitions. Prepare to challenge your muscles, conquer plateaus, and revolutionize your fitness trajectory with the power of blood occlusion training.

Consider this Introduction your steppingstone into this world—setting the scope, addressing initial uncertainties, and igniting the curiosity to delve deeper. The following chapters will build upon this groundwork, equipping you with the knowledge to implement BOT into your fitness regime and to understand its underlying mechanisms and benefits in detail.

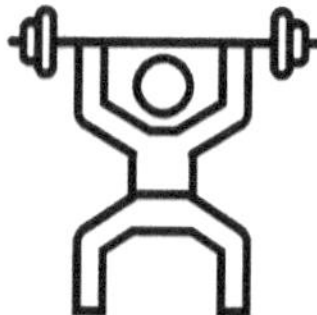

Chapter 1

The Foundations of Muscle Mastery

Embarking on a quest for muscle mastery can be an exhilarating journey, but it's imperative to lay a strong foundation before diving into the nuanced realms of growth and conditioning. For those aiming to sculpt their physique without dedicating endless hours to lifting gargantuan weights, there is a compelling cutting-edge science at your fingertips. It is the concept of blood occlusion training (BOT), an innovative and scientifically backed method that promises potent results through the strategic restriction of blood flow. BOT does not just promise change — it delivers, by triggering an anabolic response that can lead to significant muscle gain while using lighter loads (Loenneke et al., 2012). This may seem counterintuitive but think of it as a lesser-known cheat code to muscle growth. In this chapter, we will firmly plant our feet on the grounds of muscle building's basic tenets, ensuring a robust understanding of muscle hypertrophy. From there, we will dip our toes into the waters of blood occlusion training, setting the stage for a transformative approach to fitness that appeals to athletes, military personnel, the elderly, bodybuilders, and the injured alike.

The Science Behind Muscle Growth

Understanding muscle growth is essential for anyone looking to build a strong, athletic physique. Muscle growth, or hypertrophy, occurs when muscle fibers undergo damage through intense physical activity, triggering a repair process that results in larger and stronger muscles (Schoenfeld, 2010). To comprehend this transformative process fully, we must delve into the types of muscle fibers and the role they play.

There are primarily two types of muscle fibers: Type I, known as slow-twitch fibers, and Type II, or fast-twitch fibers. Type I fibers are endurance-oriented and more resistant to fatigue, while Type II fibers provide strength and power but fatigue more quickly. Different training modalities can target these specific fiber types, but all muscle fibers have the potential for growth when subjected to the right stimuli (Fry, 2004).

When we lift weights or engage in resistance training, we create microscopic tears in our muscle fibers. This damage signals the body to initiate a repair process, involving the fusion of muscle cells, known as satellite cells, to the damaged fibers, thereby increasing their size and capacity (Charge & Rudnicki, 2004). This process requires adequate nutrition and rest to be effective.

The addition of blood occlusion training (BOT), an innovative method, adds a new dimension to muscle growth strategies. Occlusion training involves the application of pressure to a limb during low-intensity resistance training. This pressure limits blood flow to the working muscles, creating a hypoxic environment which causes an accumulation of metabolites and stimulates muscle growth, analogous to high-intensity training effects, but with lighter weights (Loenneke et al., 2012).

Importantly, BOT has been shown to preferentially target Type II muscle fibers, despite the use of low-load resistance which normally targets Type I fibers. This suggests that BOT can trigger an anabolic response akin to heavy lifting, making it a valuable tool for a range of individuals, from athletes to the elderly, who may not be able to handle heavy weights due to injury or other limitations (Loenneke et al., 2010).

For muscle fibers to grow, they need three primary things: mechanical tension, metabolic stress, and muscle damage. Mechanical tension involves the force placed on muscles during exercise, metabolic stress is related to the build-up of metabolites like lactate, and muscle damage is caused by exerting muscles beyond what they are accustomed to. BOT effectively induces metabolic stress, potentially reducing the need for muscle damage and mechanical tension traditionally achieved through heavy lifting (Scott et al., 2015).

Growth factors also play a crucial role in muscle development. These include hormones like IGF-1, which help promote an anabolic environment conducive to muscle growth. By restricting blood flow and then releasing that pressure, BOT may cause a surge of growth hormone release, further enhancing the anabolic process (Takarada et al., 2000).

Nutrition is another critical element in muscle growth. Protein synthesis must exceed protein breakdown for hypertrophy to occur. Consuming sufficient protein, particularly after a workout, provides the necessary amino acids for muscle repair and growth. Additionally, carbohydrates help replenish glycogen stores and also release insulin, a hormone that further supports anabolic processes (Phillips & Van Loon, 2011).

Recovery is just as important as the training itself in the muscle growth equation. During rest, the body repairs and strengthens muscles; without adequate recovery, the muscles cannot fully rebound and grow. Sleep, nutrition, and proper hydration all contribute to effective recovery.

Blood flow is essential for delivering nutrients to muscles and removing waste products. By temporarily restricting blood flow using BOT, followed by its restoration, there is a rapid influx of blood that can help in the nutrient delivery and waste removal process, potentially speeding up recovery and allowing for quicker muscle growth (Loenneke & Pujol, 2009).

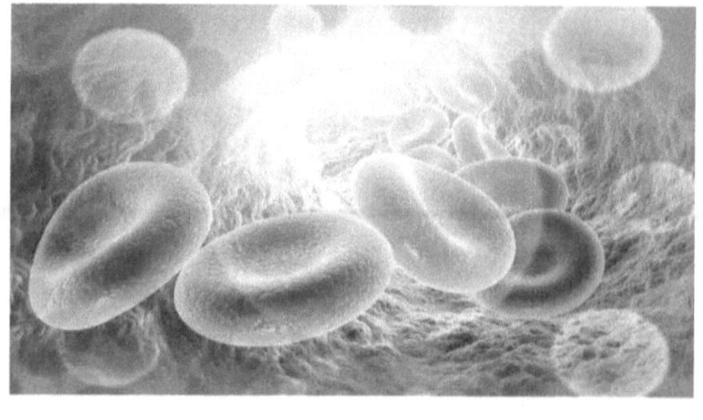 It is also important to understand that muscle growth is not a linear process. Plateaus are common, and that's where different training techniques, like BOT, come in handy. They provide new stimuli to muscles, tricking them into continued growth by altering the stressors during a workout (Suga et al., 2012).

While BOT is an effective tool, it should be part of a holistic approach to fitness, which includes conventional strength training, cardiovascular activities, and flexibility exercises. Combining BOT with traditional methods can lead to a well-rounded fitness regime that maximizes muscle growth.

Finally, individual variability plays a role in muscle growth. Genetics, age, hormone levels, and lifestyle choices all affect how muscles respond to training. Recognizing this, BOT can be tailored to suit individual needs and capabilities, ensuring safe and effective workouts for diverse populations.

Understanding the science of muscle growth is pivotal for developing a sophisticated and effective workout regimen. With the knowledge of muscle fibers, the stimuli required for growth, the impact of blood flow, and the integration of BOT, individuals can work smarter, not just harder, to achieve their fitness and muscle-building goals.

In conclusion, muscle mastery is not achieved overnight. It is a complex process informed by biology and can be significantly enhanced by applying the principles of blood occlusion training. Integrating these insights will pave the way for impressive, sustainable muscle growth and overall fitness.

Understanding Blood Occlusion Training: The Basics

Blood Occlusion Training (BOT), or blood flow restriction (BFR) training as some may know it, may sound like a technique reserved for elite athletes or hardcore bodybuilders. However, this powerful and scientifically proven method offers surprising benefits for a wide array of individuals seeking strength gains or muscle recovery. Dive into the essentials of BOT and discover how it might just revolutionize your fitness routine.

At its core, BOT involves the application of a tourniquet around the limb being worked out, either the upper arms or legs. There are different types of tourniquets, such as a medical-grade tourniquet, an elastic quick-release tourniquet (shown), plain elastic wraps, etc. The tourniquet or wrap can come in different widths and sizes; it comes down to personal preference, what feels comfortable yet still gets the job done. You can easily find a variety of blood occlusion training wraps or tourniquets by searching on Amazon. Give a few different options a try!

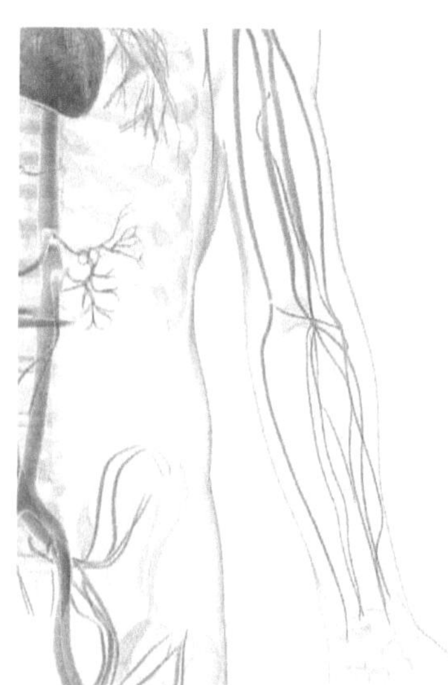

The whole idea is not to cut off blood supply entirely, but rather to restrict the venous return of blood from the muscle while maintaining arterial blood flow to the muscle. This creates a local environment within the muscles that favors growth, even while using much lighter weights than one might in a traditional workout.

The tourniquet's pressure is key; it must be precise, enough to occlude the veins but not so much that it stops arterial inflow. That is why proper technique and sometimes even clinical supervision are imperative for newbies to BOT. But when done correctly, you can reap the benefits using only about 20% of your one-repetition maximum weight during exercise—a feature that makes BOT particularly appealing to various groups.

Athletes looking to gain a competitive edge can integrate BOT into their training to enhance muscle strength and size without overloading the joints. For fitness enthusiasts aiming to bulk up for a show or fast-track their muscle gains, the efficiency of BOT is unmatched. But it is not just for the young and fit; the elderly can safely use BOT to maintain muscle mass, which is crucial for mobility and overall health.

Those who have sustained injuries also stand to gain from BOT, as its low-resistance nature lends itself well to rehabilitation. Without the need for heavy lifting, recovery from injuries like ACL tears, ankle sprains, and patellofemoral syndrome becomes less daunting. BOT can even be a game-changer for amputees who cannot lift heavy weights like before and are seeking to build strength for prosthetic limb use.

The military community, too, may find BOT beneficial for both wounded soldiers in recovery and those looking to maintain peak physical condition without the added stress of high-resistance training. It helps bridge the gap between injury and return to duty by fostering muscle growth when traditional training methods are not feasible.

Highly trained athletes, particularly those suffering from conditions such as muscle strains, ACL and meniscus tears, stress fractures, etc. can tailor BOT to their fitness routine, enhancing strength without exacerbating their condition. For all these groups, the ability to stimulate muscle hypertrophy at a fraction of the load normally required provides a unique and effective alternative to traditional high-load training.

However, safety in BOT must be a top priority. A set of criteria ensures that the training is not only effective but also harmless. These safety criteria include having a Body Mass Index (BMI) less than 30 kg/m², no known risk factors for thromboembolism, an absence of peripheral vascular disease, no pregnant women and no uncontrolled hypertension.

Further safety measures stipulate that those individuals with a history of cerebral hemorrhage, ischemic heart diseases, and severe aortic stenosis should steer clear of BOT. It is also wise to consult a healthcare professional before starting BOT, especially if you fall into one of the higher-risk categories or are new to the practice.

It is important to emphasize that while BOT can seem intimidating at first glance, when done responsibly, it is a safe and highly effective technique. It has been widely researched and is supported by a growing body of evidence pointing to its efficacy (Loenneke et al., 2012). Personal trainers and therapists trained in BOT can provide guidance on the correct band placement, pressure levels, and exercise routines to ensure both safety and effectiveness.

You might wonder if BOT really can replace traditional heavy lifting for muscle gains—and the answer is nuanced. For certain outcomes and benefits, particularly for those who cannot or should not lift heavy, BOT can indeed mimic the physiological muscle stress typically achieved with heavier weights (Cook et al., 2014).

But that does not mean it is for everyone or every situation. The brilliance of BOT lies in its versatility and applicability to diverse populations. It is not meant to entirely replace conventional strength training but to complement it or serve as an alternative when circumstances demand.

To sum up, Blood Occlusion Training opens up a new frontier in physical conditioning and muscle mastery. Its scientifically-backed methodology offers a path for many—athletes, the elderly, the recovering, and others—to achieve significant fitness gains with a lower risk of injury. It is less about the weight and more about the technique, offering a compelling strategy for those looking to push their limits in a new and safe

way.

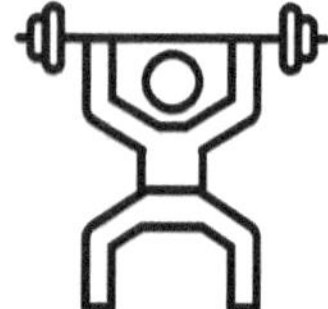

The Science Behind Blood Occlusion Training

Diving deeper into our journey, Chapter 2 explores the ingenious science that catalyzes muscle growth through blood occlusion training (BOT). It is a technique that is a bit of a fitness hack, seemingly deceiving your body into believing it is pushing heavier weights. By partially restricting blood flow with strategically placed wraps or cuffs, BOT triggers metabolic stress and muscle hypertrophy, akin to that produced by traditional high-load resistance training—yet it does so with much lighter weights (Loenneke et al., 2012). This means potentially less strain on joints and connective tissues, which is great news for those recovering from injuries or with physical limitations. The restricted blood flow is not just about increasing the burn; there is a cascade of physiological events from hormonal responses to cellular swelling that amplify muscle growth (Suga et al., 2012). Grounded in the principles of kaatsu training, a technique originating in Japan, BOT manipulates the body's natural repair systems and accelerates muscle building by inducing a state of localized hypoxia, thereby taxing the slow-twitch muscle fibers and rapidly recruiting the explosive fast-twitch fibers more typical of heavyweight lifting (Abe et al., 2006). It is like packing the effects of an intensive, time-consuming workout into a session that is gentler on your body and respectful of your precious time.

How Blood Occlusion Builds REAL Muscle

In understanding the impressive muscular adaptations brought about by blood occlusion training (BOT), also known as blood flow restriction (BFR) training, we are not diving into some trend of the moment—we are talking about a solid, scientifically-backed method that enables real muscle growth even with lower intensity workouts. This technique,

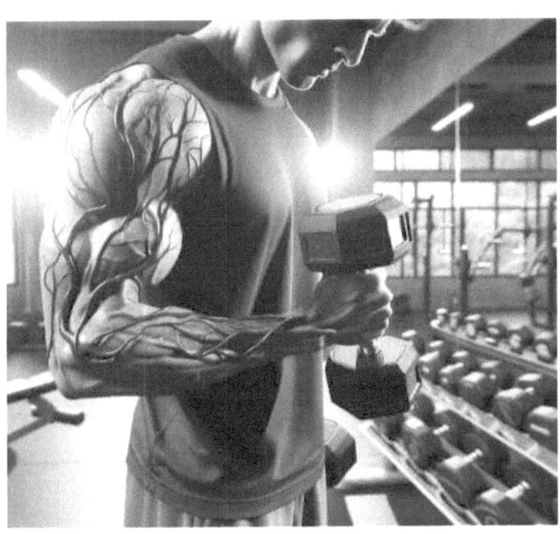

somewhat reminiscent of an ancient warrior binding their limbs before a battle, harnesses the body's physiological response to strategically applied

pressure, inducing an environment ripe for muscle

hypertrophy. But what exactly transpires in the muscles

during blood occlusion training? Let us dissect the

science beneath the surface.

Blood occlusion training (BOT), represents a

fascinating synthesis of exercise science and practical

know-how, resulting in a potent stimulus for muscle

strength and hypertrophy. While it might seem

counterintuitive, the underlying mechanisms behind

BOT are grounded in a robust physiological framework.

To kick things off, BOT requires the application of a

restrictive device – it could be a specialized blood

pressure cuff, a medical tourniquet, or even knee and

wrist wraps – snugly wrapped around the limb just

proximal to the muscle you are targeting. What this

does is modulate the blood flow, particularly curbing

the venous return from the muscle while maintaining

arterial blood flow into the muscle (Loenneke et al.,

2012).

This partial blood flow restriction creates a low-

oxygen environment within the muscle, which is where

the magic begins. When muscles are deprived of

oxygen, they respond by recruiting larger, fast-twitch

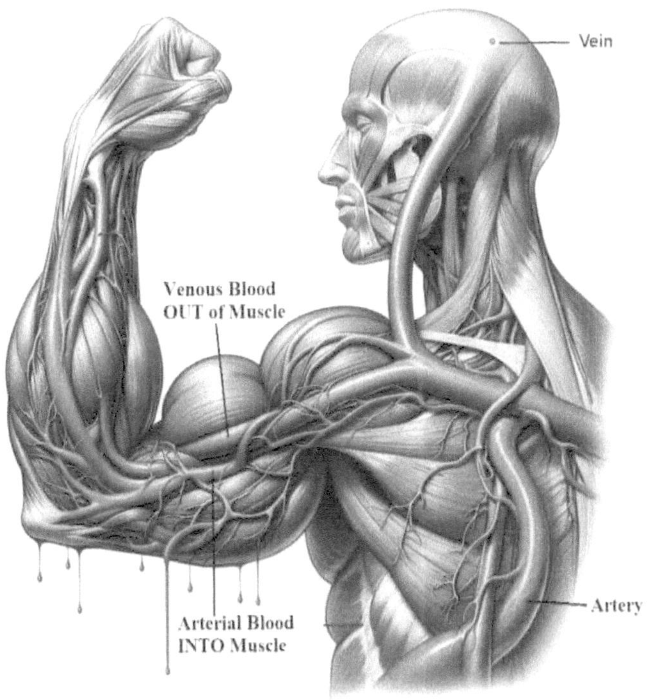

muscle fibers much earlier than they would under normal conditions. This recruitment pattern is similar to what is observed with high-intensity workouts – typically associated with muscle growth and increased strength (Loenneke et al., 2012).

What is especially interesting about this technique is that it allows these fibers to be recruited at significantly lighter weights than would normally be required. This means less stress on joints and connective tissues, which can be a boon for those with injuries, older populations, or even athletes who are recovering from strenuous training sessions or injuries as well.

Metabolic accumulation stands at the cornerstone of BOT. Rather than allowing the metabolic byproducts of exercise to dissipate, occlusion creates an environment where these substances are retained near the muscles. This local milieu, rich in metabolites, fosters a surge in anabolic growth factors. Picture the metabolic buildup like a party where all the important muscle-building guests stay longer, mingling and enhancing the growth potential within the muscle tissue.

As the exercise continues, metabolites such as lactate start to accumulate. This buildup is crucial, as it is believed to be a key driver in the muscle growth process by stimulating growth hormone release, increasing protein synthesis, and activating satellite cells, which are essential for repairing and building muscle tissue (Fujita et al., 2007).

Lactate often dismissed as merely a fatigue-inducing byproduct, lactate accumulation actually acts as a trigger for an astonishing growth hormone surge (Takarada et al., 2000). Imagine an increase of 290 times above baseline! To put that into perspective, traditional heavy resistance training without occlusion typically manages only half of this hormonal rally. It is the equivalent of swapping a regular shot of espresso for a caffeine boost that launches you into orbit. Growth hormone is critically involved in tissue repair and muscle growth, rendering it a pivotal player in BOT's effectiveness.

Another contributing factor is the acute muscle cell swelling that occurs during BOT. Think of it as a localized muscle pump where increased pressure forces plasma into muscle cells, which in turn are equipped with sensors detecting this change in volume. This cellular stretch is like a secret handshake telling the muscle to grow (Loenneke et al., 2012). The restriction of venous return causes fluid to accumulate within the muscle, which, in cellular terms, can be read as a threat to the integrity of the cell. The cell's response to this 'swelling' is a muscle-building one, reinforcing the cellular structure to accommodate the increased fluid (Schoenfeld, 2013). This swelling, or "muscle pump," may also act as an anabolic signal in its own right, contributing to the overall hypertrophic response of the muscle. Furthermore, the mechanical tension created along with metabolic stress sparks a delightful cascade of muscle-building signals within the body.

The hypoxia – or lack of oxygen – induced by the blood flow restriction also plays a role. This state stimulates the production of vascular endothelial growth factor (VEGF), which is involved in the formation of new blood vessels, enhancing the muscle's ability to receive nutrients and oxygen in the long run (Manini & Clark, 2009).

Another fascinating aspect is the decreased expression of atrogenes. These genes, with their role in muscle atrophy, become less active under occlusion. Hence, BOT not only encourages growth but puts the brakes on the loss of muscle mass (Fujita et al., 2007). It is akin to having one foot firmly on the growth accelerator while easing off the attrition pedal. In continuation, BOT also appears to reduce muscle protein breakdown during and after workouts, potentially due to the sustained increase in insulin-like growth factor-1 (IGF-1) levels, further tilting the muscle metabolism towards growth (Manini & Clark, 2009).

Further underpinning the effectiveness of BOT is the role of satellite cells. These cells act as muscle repair agents and when proliferation is stimulated via occlusion training, muscle protein synthesis kicks into high gear. Satellite cell activation ramps up mTOR signaling, an essential pathway that governs muscle protein synthesis, and also boosts NOS-1 expression, enhancing nutrient delivery and growth factor production (Fujita et al., 2007). The BOT environment, therefore, becomes a fertile ground for muscle regeneration and growth.

Another bio-advantage of BOT is the reduction in myostatin concentrations. You can consider myostatin as the chaperone that tries to keep muscle growth in check—by reducing its influence, BOT effectively unleashes the potential for greater muscle gains (Laurentino et al., 2012).

Moreover, the recruitment of Type 2 fibers, often associated with high-load exercises, is yet another benefit of BOT. Under occlusion, even when using lighter weights, these power-packed fibers spring into action much earlier in the exercise set. It is like tricking the body into believing it is hefting heavier weights, without the associated stress on joints and tissues (Abe et al., 2006).

It is not all about muscle, though; BOT can also positively affect the tendons. Due to the increased collagen synthesis that occurs as a response to the restricted blood flow, tendons can become stronger and more resilient. This effect enhances overall limb stability and can contribute to long-term joint health.

Integrating all these mechanisms, blood occlusion training excels in crafting a physical landscape where muscles can grow more efficiently and effectively. It is important to note that while these processes seem focused on biology and chemistry, their outcomes are hugely practical. Athletes, military personnel, amputees, bodybuilders, and even those recovering from injuries or the elderly, can witness significant gains in muscle size and strength without the need for high-intensity loads.

So why does this matter? For anyone seeking to optimize their fitness routine, understanding that BOT is more than a fad—it is a nuanced approach that flips the script of traditional muscle-building doctrine. By leveraging the body's own biochemical processes in a novel way, BOT can supplement or even replace conventional heavy lifting, making it an invaluable tool for those intent on getting fast, real fitness results.

As we continue weaving through the tapestry of blood occlusion training, it becomes abundantly clear that this technique is anchored in hard science with impressive results. The interplay of lactate, growth hormones, cellular swelling, gene expression, satellite cells, myostatin reduction, and fiber recruitment all combines to transform the body in a profound way. It is truly a method that speaks to the saying 'work smarter, not harder,' giving your muscles the intense experience they need to grow, without the heavy toll.

Evidence also suggests that the benefits of BOT extend beyond the immediate response to training. Long-term adaptations have been observed, including increased muscle cross-sectional area and muscle strength, demonstrating that the effects of BOT are not merely transient pump but constitute substantial muscle conditioning (Takarada et al., 2000).

It is interesting to note, too, that BOT can evoke systemic effects. Although the restriction is applied locally, the hormonal milieu created by the local hypertrophic response has the potential to influence muscle growth in non-restricted muscles as well. This is a huge benefit!

Of course, like any training regimen, progression and adaptation are part of the journey. Initially, one might find the perceived exertion during BOT to be greater than traditional training methods, as the body adapts to the unusual stimuli. However, over time, this sensation diminishes as the body becomes more efficient at dealing with the hypoxic conditions and clearing accumulated metabolites. As the saying goes, " no pain, no gain!"

Finally, it is worth considering the psychological aspects of training. BOT can afford individuals a novel and accessible method to experience intense resistance training benefits without the intimidation of heavy loads. This psychological edge could motivate those who might otherwise abstain from traditional strength training, due to the reduced mechanical strain and relative ease of execution.

In conclusion, BOT represents a relatively new but scientifically sound approach that enables individuals to optimize muscle growth and strength using low-intensity exercise. It has opened up pathways for diverse populations to experience the benefits of resistance training while minimizing the risk of injury and strain on the musculoskeletal system (Takarada et al., 2000; Loenneke et al., 2012).

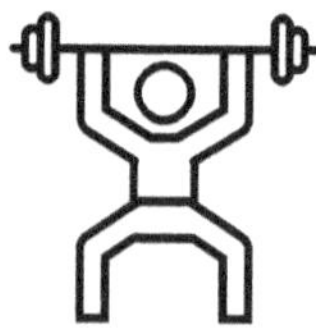

Chapter 3

Methods and Procedures

oving forward from the essential understanding of blood occlusion training (BOT) and its scientific rationale, we navigate the landscape of implementation in "Methods and Procedures". This pivotal chapter lays down the practical blueprint for executing BOT with precision and safety. As we delve into the specifics, you will learn to tailor the protocols to suit diverse fitness landscapes, covering the needs of pro athletes to the rehabilitating injured. Our discourse pivots around meticulously illustrating how to calibrate pressure and discern the Goldilocks zone—a balance critical for invoking optimized stress without overstepping into harm's territory. Nuanced guidance paves the way for accessing the potential of BOT across varying physical exigencies, ensuring every individual—be it a soldier in training or a gym enthusiast—extracts the quintessential benefits that this transformative method promises (Patterson & Brandner, 2018).

Specific Blood Occlusion Training Protocols for Athletes, Injured, and Military Personnel

Blood occlusion training (BOT) may seem like a secret weapon shrouded in gym lore, but it is grounded in solid science. Athletes, military personnel, and those recovering from musculoskeletal injuries can all benefit from this technique, which allows for significant strength gains with minimal equipment and lower weights. Let us dive into the specific protocols that can lead to rapid muscle growth and recovery.

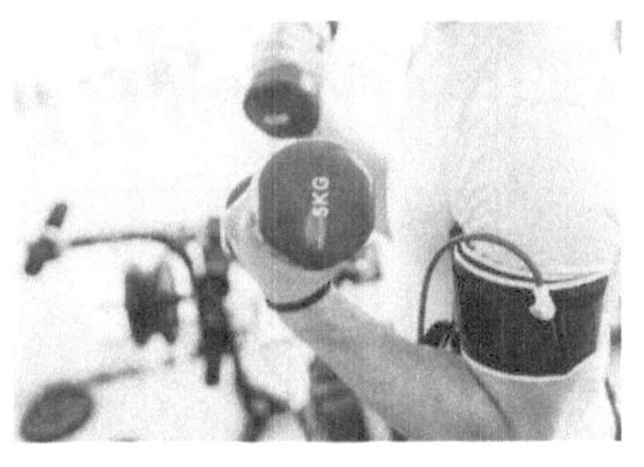

First and foremost, it is essential to understand the placement of the tourniquet. Whether you are working out the upper or lower body, the tourniquet should be positioned as high on the limb as possible.

For the arms, wrap just under the shoulder joint,

targeting the biceps. For the legs, place the wrap right

below the gluteal fold close to the groin. These

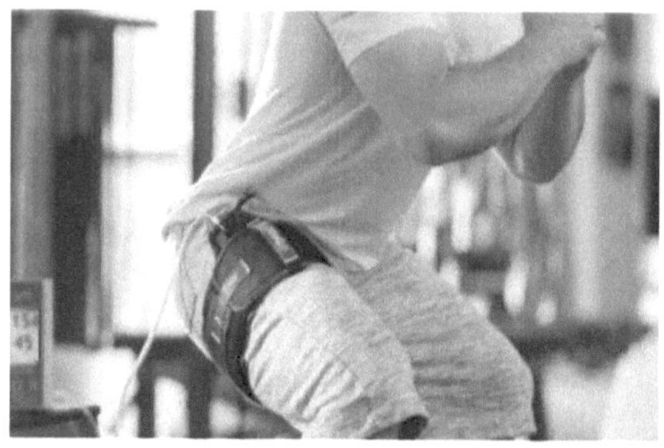 placement strategies are key for maximizing blood flow restriction

while minimizing risks. No other placement is

recommended; only apply the tourniquet to the upper

arms and legs. This positioning is sufficient to induce a

systemic response. While the blood restriction is

localized, the hormonal changes caused by the

hypertrophic response in the restricted area can also

influence muscle growth in non-restricted muscles.

This is truly remarkable!

The tightness of the tourniquet is a delicate balance. The perceived tightness should be about 7 on a scale of 10, which equates to 70% occlusion. It is critical to get this right. If you are in pain before even starting your exercises, or if you cannot complete the planned repetitions, the wrap is too tight. The objective is to restrict venous blood flow without severely limiting arterial influx.

Regarding the actual lifting protocol, athletes and those in recovery should begin with 30 repetitions of an exercise at 20-30% of their one-rep max (1RM). This initial set should be followed by three sets of 15 repetitions with a short 30-second rest in between. This workload is designed to induce hypertrophy without placing undue strain on recovering or fatigued muscles (Lixandrão et al., 2018).

For the frequency, incorporating this protocol into your routine 2-3 times a week seems to strike the right balance between stimulation and recovery. It is vital for athletes, particularly those in season or under operational demands, to avoid over-training, which can hinder performance and increase the likelihood of injury.

Military personnel, often on strict schedules and with varying levels of physical readiness, can incorporate BOT to maintain or increase strength despite limitations on equipment and time. This can be particularly useful in deployment scenarios or when access to traditional training facilities is prohibitive (Cook et al., 2014).

In the case of injured individuals, particularly post-op musculoskeletal surgery patients, BOT is not merely a means of muscle building; it is a crucial element in preserving muscle mass and strength during periods of lowered activity. A healthcare professional must monitor the application, but the benefits of BOT in accelerating rehabilitation cannot be overstated (Patterson & Brandner, 2017).

Another consideration is the implementation of dynamic exercises versus static holds within the BOT framework. For athletes focusing on explosive power, dynamic movements under occlusion provide an excellent stimulus. Similarly, those rehabbing injuries might find static holds beneficial in the initial stages to reintroduce strain to healing tissues.

Moreover, while repetition and set structure is important, so is the exercise selection. For the upper body, the beginner exercises would be bicep curls and tricep extensions. For the lower body, the exercises would be seated leg extensions and hamstring curls.

First, master these beginner exercises with the appropriate tourniquet tightness before moving onto other exercises. In the following chapters, we will discuss advancing the blood occlusion exercises once the basics are complete. Compound movements versus isolation exercises can elicit different responses under occlusion, providing targeted improvements relevant to specific athletic or rehabilitative needs. However, the basics need to be met in order to get that perfect recipe for success and elicit the BOT response.

As with any training regimen, warming up becomes doubly significant when incorporating BOT to safeguard against strain or further injury. A pre-occlusion warm-up should aim to increase tissue temperature and blood flow to the muscles that will be trained.

Cooling down and recovery are just as crucial in the BOT methodology. Further details on this subject will be provided in subsequent chapters. However, after releasing the tourniquet, it is wise to follow up with low-intensity exercises and stretching to promote blood flow and enhance recovery—especially given the localized stress that BOT places on muscle tissues (Loenneke et al., 2012).

Regular evaluation is also a part of the BOT process. Athletes and military personnel should assess their progress both in terms of subjective feeling and objective measures like girth and dynamometry to ensure that the BOT is contributing positively to their strength and muscle growth goals without causing undue fatigue or injury.

For both athletes and military personnel, ensuring the tourniquet is applied using the suitable material is of the essence. While commercial products are available, ensuring that any DIY approach does not damage the tissue or create too much discomfort is crucial. Elastic wraps should be the material of choice when commercial options are not accessible.

Finally, athletes and others engaged in BOT must stay hydrated and maintain a diet adequate in protein to support the increased demands on the muscle repair system. Nutrition and hydration are integral to optimizing the results from BOT, much like with traditional strength training.

In conclusion, blood occlusion training offers a promising solution to gain strength and maintain muscle without the wear and tear of heavy lifting. By following these protocols and considerations, athletes, military personnel, and the injured can achieve their fitness and rehabilitation goals effectively. Adopting

BOT into one's routine requires precision, caution, and

a willingness to adapt, but the potential to improve

physical capacity is significant.

Proven Scientific Case Studies

In the previous chapters, we have laid the groundwork for understanding blood occlusion training (BOT) and explored its underlying mechanisms. Now it is time to delve into the scientific evidence supporting the efficacy of this innovative training method. We will examine notable case studies that highlight the benefits of BOT, especially in comparison to traditional training regimens.

Five significant case studies were found that had at least a blood occlusion training group and a regular exercise group or a control group. The authors of these studies reported findings that blood occlusion training does increase strength and decrease atrophy more than the alternative high intensity training, regular exercise, or no training at all.

One groundbreaking study that sets the stage for blood occlusion's merits involved participants who incorporated low-load resistance muscular training during moderate restriction of blood flow is an effective exercise for early muscular training after reconstruction of the anterior cruciate ligament. These results strongly indicate the benefit of implementing a blood flow occlusion training program to the healthy, post-op patient who underwent a sport related musculoskeletal surgery to increase strength and return to prior level of function more efficiently and without damage to the healing structures (Takayama et al., 2015). The authors deduced that this method fosters early muscle strength gains, which is incredibly beneficial for patients recovering from such invasive surgeries. This finding is a nod to BOT's potential in accelerating the rehabilitation timeline.

After comparing blood occlusion training to regular exercise, researchers agreed blood occlusion training would be beneficial for patients that want to increase muscle size and strength. Studies show blood occlusion training is an effective exercise for early muscular training after surgery. However, these studies used healthy patients; therefore, it is not acceptable to use blood occlusion training on patients with cardiovascular diseases or other health concerns. Physical therapists can use blood occlusion training with the known specific protocols found in these studies to help rehabilitate healthy adults after a reconstruction surgery to get them back to prior level of function.

Another study concluded that the multiple sets of low-intensity resistance exercise with blood flow restriction could achieve the same metabolic stress as multiple sets of high-intensity resistance exercise without blood flow restriction (Ohta et al., 2003). The authors concluded that low intensity exercise with blood flow restriction is an efficient and effective method of maintaining and/or increasing post-surgical muscle size and knee function, superior to traditional exercise alone (Sato et al., 2005). This is a revelation for those looking to achieve the benefits of intense workouts without the associated wear and tear. This also affirms BOT's role in not just muscle preservation but also in proactive strength building without heavy lifting.

In another compelling investigation, the results showed that blood flow restriction applied in intervals to an immobilized, bedridden group showed an increase in muscle strength and thigh/leg circumference after 16 weeks. The author's concluded that repetitive, interval-applied blood flow restriction to the lower extremity prevents disuse muscular weakness, which shows the importance and benefit of blood flow restriction even when not paired with exercise (Abe et al., 2006). This finding is mind blowing!!

Physical therapists are increasingly drawing on these findings to inform their practices. By adapting specific BOT protocols, they can support their patients in not only recovering from surgeries but also in achieving a return to pre-injury function levels and prevent muscle breakdown with bedridden patients (Patterson et al., 2019).

While these studies illuminate the efficacy of BOT, it is critical to recognize that more inquiries are essential for a complete understanding of its implications, especially concerning cardiovascular impacts. Health professionals must tread cautiously and prioritize patient safety and suitability for BOT. It is imperative to note, while BOT shows promise, its application must be carefully considered. These individuals in these studies did not have any diagnosed cardiovascular conditions, reinforcing the importance of appropriately screening patients before implementing BOT. By following the established procedures from the aforementioned studies, practitioners can look to achieve predictable and beneficial outcomes for their patients.

In conclusion, the evidence in favor of BOT is compelling, with repeated demonstrations of its superiority in fostering muscle growth and strength, particularly after surgical interventions. This segment of our journey through the BOT landscape verifies the method's value and sets the stage for its application across diverse scenarios.

It is worth noting that future studies are required to optimize protocols further, tailor applications for specific populations, and confirm long-term safety. For now, BOT stands as a scientifically backed approach, encouraging those in the worlds of fitness, rehabilitation, and beyond to embrace a method that maximizes results while minimizing strain.

As we move forward into the upcoming chapters, we will build on this foundation of empirical evidence, exploring BOT's extended applications and the path to mastery for various users, including athletes and specialized populations.

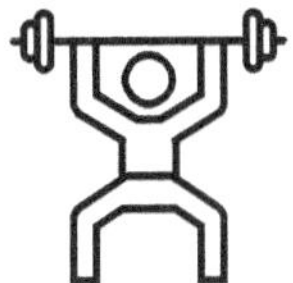

Chapter 4

Blood Occlusion for Special Populations

In delving into blood occlusion training (BOT), we have explored the science and protocols suitable for various athletic and rehabilitation contexts. Now, it is time to tailor this potent training methodology for those who typically sit outside the usual fitness paradigms—special populations. In this chapter, we will examine how age, unique health considerations, and distinctive physiological needs factor into adapting BOT for maximum efficacy and safety. Special focus is given to the elderly, who can reap substantial benefits from the gentler, subtler stress that BOT places on the body, stimulating muscle growth and enhancing circulation without the high-impact risks associated with traditional resistance training (Patterson & Brandner, 2017). Precise considerations will be addressed, ensuring that blood flow restriction training can be safely integrated into the fitness repertoire of individuals who might otherwise face contraindications for standard high-intensity exercises. Aligning with best practices, our guidance is backed by recent research that sheds light on suitable pressures, duration, and frequency for various special populations, setting the stage for a transformative yet safe training experience (Loenneke et al., 2012).

Adapting BOT for the Elderly

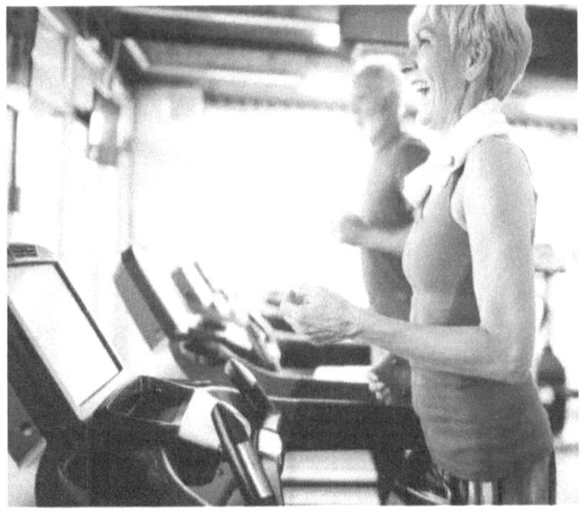

As we dig into the nuances of Blood Occlusion Training (BOT) for special populations, a particularly important demographic to consider is the elderly. One paramount concern in older adults is the natural decline in muscle mass and strength—a condition known as sarcopenia. This loss can greatly diminish quality of life and increase the risk of falls and fractures. Weightlifting, often the go-to approach for muscle building, may not always be feasible for older individuals due to joint stress and other health concerns. This is where the brilliance of BOT steps in, offering a scientifically sound workaround.

Theology aside, the crux of BOT's appeal to older populations hinges on its low-intensity approach paired with substantial gains in muscle strength and size. So, let us dissect the specifics of an elderly protocol and unpack the proof of its effectiveness.

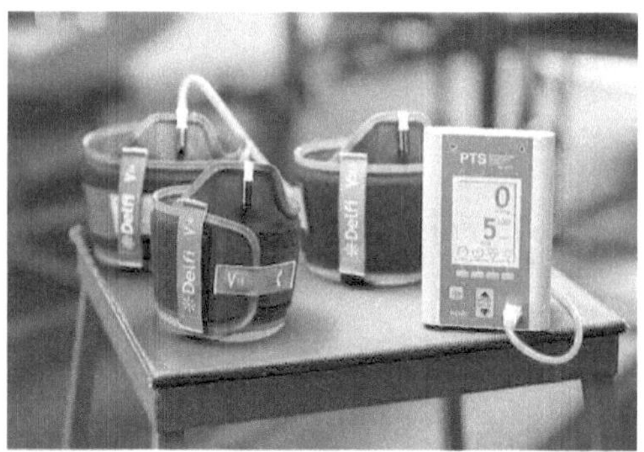

In a pioneering study, a protocol was designed for an active elderly group to perform 20-minute treadmill walking sessions at a speed of 2.5 miles per hour (Mph), five days per week, for a duration of six weeks. During these sessions, a calculated restriction pressure between 160 to 200 mm

Hg was applied to both legs using a blood pressure (BP) cuff for the entirety of each session (Patterson & Brandner, 2018). Such restriction benchmarks are critical since they ensure safety while also promoting sufficient metabolic stress necessary for muscle adaptation.

So, why this particular protocol? For starters, walking is a functional, low-impact exercise that most elderly individuals can perform without significant risk. The speed of 2.5 Mph is brisk yet manageable, helping to maintain cardiovascular health without overexertion. And importantly, the blood occlusion element serves to enhance what would be modest gains from walking alone. This technique of blood occlusion paired with walking, would also benefit amputees looking to enhance their strength. Amputees would be able to walk with their prosthetic leg in a low impact setting and reap the rewards. BOT would get them the most efficient way of gaining "high intensity-like" muscle without picking up a single weight.

But does it work? Indeed, it does. The proof is in the outcomes.

The study highlighted those participants who adhered to the 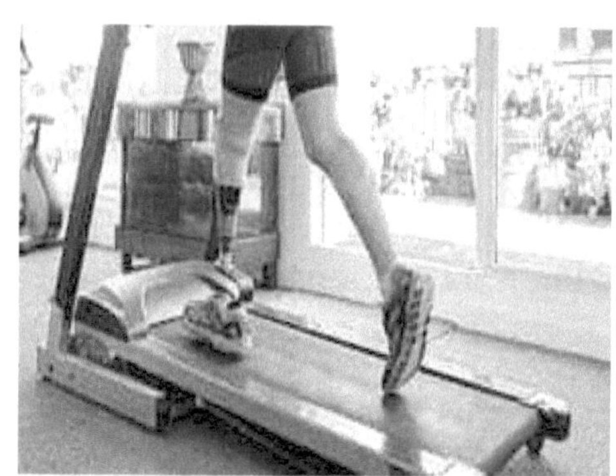 blood occlusion-walking routine experienced considerable increases in knee extension and flexion strength. Essentially, this means that the muscles enabling participants to kick out and draw in their legs grew stronger—an essential aspect of functional mobility (Patterson & Brandner, 2018).

Furthermore, the muscle-bone cross-sectional area saw an uptick. In layman's terms, the diameter of the thigh where the muscles and bones lie became more pronounced—a signifier of improved musculoskeletal health. This is a crucial change, as it implies enhanced support and stability for the leg and, therefore; body (Patterson et al., 2019).

Participants did not just gain raw strength; their ultrastructural muscle changes were also noted via ultrasound-estimated skeletal muscle mass improvements. Visualize the structural integrity of muscle fibers getting a boost—something we would typically expect from heavy lifting yet achieved here with walking and occlusion (Patterson et al., 2019).

In terms of how this translated to daily life, the participants in the blood occlusion-walk group showcased an increase in functional mobility. This refers to their capacity to perform everyday activities with ease—whether that is climbing stairs, carrying groceries, or transitioning from sitting to standing.

However, the study reported no change in estimated peak oxygen uptake, a measure of cardiovascular fitness, for either the active group or the control group (Patterson et al., 2019). So, while BOT proved potent for muscular development, it did not move the needle for aerobic capacity in this context, which is to be expected since we are only walking and not putting high amounts of stress on the body. This is a vital consideration when using BOT for the older adult population, in order to conserve energy and prevent fatigue yet still grow muscle and improve functional mobility.

What is the big picture takeaway from these findings? For starters, six weeks of targeted blood occlusion-walk training can ignite significant muscle remodeling and functional improvements without necessarily targeting cardiovascular fitness. This is substantial for elderly individuals looking to maintain or even regain muscle strength and mass.

Essentially, BOT offers a training approach that is dumbed down on joint stress but ramped up in efficiency—a hybrid that sounds almost too good to be true. Yet, it is grounded in sound, peer-reviewed research, reinforcing those innovative methods can bridge the gap between the need for physical maintenance and the challenges of aging.

The implications extend beyond individual gains. As a fitness professional, understanding how to employ and adapt this method can transform the lives of our older clients. As a caregiver, introducing elderly family members to this gentle but effective form of exercise can be a game-changer in their later years.

To encapsulate, BOT may indeed be the silver bullet of resistance training alternatives for the aging population, empowering them to robustly defy the creeping limitations of time. Using science as a steadfast compass, we are ushering in a paradigm shift in elder fitness—a shift where strength and vitality are not just preserved but proliferated with every occluded step taken.

Safety Measures and Best Practices

When it comes to Blood Occlusion Training (BOT), ensuring participant safety is paramount, especially for special populations. It is crucial to understand who should and should not practice BOT. Individuals with a BMI less than 30 kg/m^2 are generally considered to be within a safer range for this type of training since a higher BMI may be associated with increased risks of cardiovascular and metabolic conditions (Lixandrao et al., 2018).

Those with risk factors for thromboembolism, such as a history of deep vein thrombosis or pulmonary embolism, must proceed with caution or entirely avoid BOT. The restriction of blood flow could potentially dislodge a thrombus, leading to serious complications (Manini & Clark, 2009).

Individuals with peripheral vascular disease should not engage in BOT due to the compromised nature of blood circulation in their limbs. Implementing occlusion could exacerbate their condition, leading to further health complications (Patterson & Brandner, 2020).

Uncontrolled hypertension (HTN) is another contraindication for BOT. The practice of blood flow restriction could potentially elevate blood pressure to dangerous levels, creating a risk for cardiovascular events (Loenneke et al., 2012).

Past cerebrovascular incidents like cerebral hemorrhage also rule out the safe practice of BOT. Increasing intracranial pressure through occlusive maneuvers could precipitate another hemorrhagic event.

Furthermore, individuals with ischemic heart disease must avoid BOT as the strain placed on the heart from restricted blood flow could lead to myocardial ischemia or infarction (Patterson & Brandner, 2020).

Severe aortic stenosis is a strict no-go for BOT. Any increase in ventricular afterload as a result of blood flow restriction could be detrimental to an already compromised flow through a stenosed aortic valve.

Pregnancy introduces a myriad of physiological changes that complicate the safety profile of BOT. Given the lack of substantial research in this area, pregnant women should abstain from this training modality to avoid unforeseen risks to both mother and child.

Assessing personal health status and risk factors is a foundational step before considering or recommending BOT. It is always advisable to consult with a healthcare professional prior to starting any new exercise regimen, especially one that includes blood flow restriction (BFR).

Aside from these health criteria, proper technique and best practices in applying BFR cuffs or bands are crucial. It is important to note that the bands should be tight enough to occlude venous return but not so tight as to completely block arterial blood flow to the muscles (Loenneke et al., 2012).

A practical method to ensure this is by using a pressure that feels like a 7 out of 10 in terms of tightness. Additionally, guidelines suggest using wider cuffs to distribute pressure more evenly over the limb, which could potentially reduce risks (Loenneke et al., 2014).

Monitoring the sensation of the limb's during exercise is essential. Any numbness, extreme discomfort, or discoloration should prompt immediate cessation of the exercise and removal of the occlusion device.

Lastly, the duration and intensity of training play an integral role in safety. Sessions should be kept relatively short (typically less than 20 minutes per muscle group) and should not push the athlete to total exhaustion.

Training protocols should be progressively adjusted, allowing the body to acclimate to the unique stressors that BOT presents. Over time, muscle endurance and strength may improve, allowing for a gradual increase in intensity and duration while maintaining a safety-first approach.

By adhering to these safety measures and best practices, individuals and practitioners can more effectively employ BOT as a means of accelerating real fitness results while prioritizing wellness and minimizing the risk of adverse events.

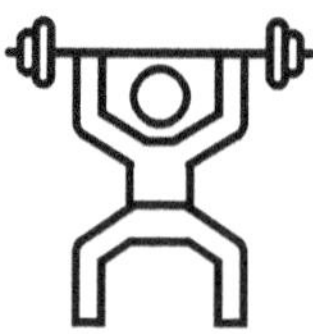

Chapter 5

Warm-up and Cool-down Techniques

In addition to the foundational safety measures and best practices with BOT, it is crucial to dive into the specifics of warm-up and cool-down techniques, which play an indispensable role in any fitness regimen or blood occlusion training program. The importance of warming up cannot be overstated—it prepares your body for the increased demand of physical activity by gradually increasing heart rate and circulation; this, in turn, loosens the joints and increases blood flow to the muscles, making them less prone to injuries (Smith, 2019). Different types of stretching, including dynamic and static stretching, serve their unique purposes. Dynamic stretches are considered most beneficial pre-workout as they help simulate the movement of the exercise itself, thereby enhancing muscular performance and reducing the risk of injury (Johnson & Johnson, 2021).

As for cooling down, this phase helps in gradually lowering the heart rate and relieves the muscles from the state of exertion experienced during the workout. This is when static stretching becomes important. Integrating flexibility exercises into your routine not only aids in injury prevention but also contributes to better muscle recovery and decreases soreness (Williams et al., 2020). This chapter will explore the mechanisms behind effective warm-up and cool-down strategies, offering insights into how these practices, when correctly integrated with blood occlusion training, can significantly enhance your fitness outcomes without the need for excessive time in the gym or lifting heavyweight. The goal here is not just about avoiding injuries but also ensuring the longevity of your fitness journey by embedding these critical practices into your daily workout regimen.

Different Types of Stretching

Transitioning smoothly from previous chapters on safety measures, it is crucial to delve into the type of stretching that not only complements your workout but enhances overall flexibility, performance, and prevents injuries. Stretching is not a one-size-fits-all affair; various methods cater to different needs, situations, and objectives. Stretching is an integral part of any fitness regimen and understanding the various types of stretching techniques can greatly enhance one's flexibility, mobility, and overall performance. Let us explore the stretching strategies that could revolutionize the way you warm up and cool down.

First up, static stretching. Static stretching involves holding a specific stretch position for a prolonged period, around 30 seconds up to two minutes. The longer the stretch is held, the greater the carryover effect in maintaining lengthening. This technique aims to lengthen and relax the muscles, making it ideal for post-workout or cool-down sessions.

By gently elongating the muscle fibers and increasing blood flow to the targeted area, static stretching helps reduce muscle tension, improve range 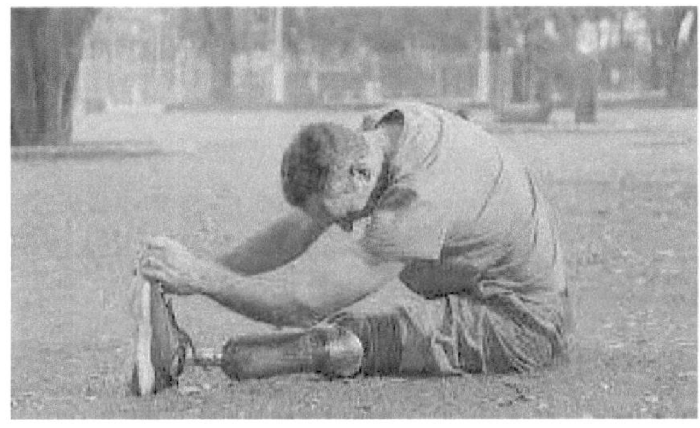 of motion, and prevent injury. It is perfect for cooling down because it helps in muscle recovery and reduces the risk of cramps and stiffness (Smith, 2019). Although once popular in warm-ups, evidence suggests that static stretching before an intense workout might actually hinder performance, suggesting its best placement at the end of your session (Johnson et al., 2012).

Dynamic stretching, on the other hand, is your go-to for warm-ups. Dynamic stretching involves moving through a series of controlled, repetitive motions that mimic the activity or sport about to be performed, gradually increasing reach, speed of movement, or both. Unlike static stretching, dynamic

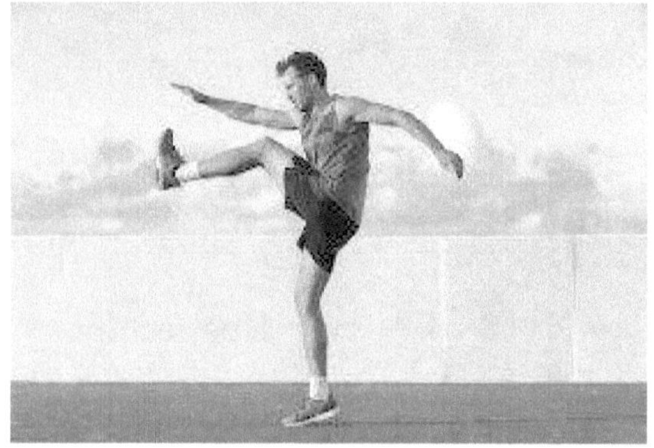

stretches are performed in a dynamic and fluid manner, gradually increasing the range of motion and warming up the muscles and joints. Dynamic stretching is particularly beneficial during warm-up routines as it helps activate the nervous system, improve circulation, and prepare the body for the specific movements and demands of the upcoming activity. Common dynamic stretches include leg swings, arm circles, and walking lunges. These movements increase blood flow and prepare your body for the physical activity ahead, essentially "waking up" the muscles in a way that is beneficial for both strength and endurance activities (Sanders, 2020).

Proprioceptive Neuromuscular Facilitation (PNF) stretching is an advanced stretching technique that combines passive stretching with isometric contractions to improve flexibility and neuromuscular control. PNF techniques typically involve stretching a muscle to its limit, then contracting the muscle against resistance for a few seconds before relaxing and stretching again. This cycle of contraction and relaxation is repeated several times, allowing for greater gains in flexibility and range of motion. PNF stretching is often used in rehabilitation settings to improve joint stability, restore muscle function, and enhance overall athletic performance.

Myofascial release is another form of stretching, though it involves using tools like foam rollers or massage balls. This is not stretching in the traditional sense but instead focuses on reducing tension and improving flexibility in the fascia, the connective tissue surrounding muscles. Especially beneficial as part of a cool-down routine, it helps in muscle recovery and reducing soreness (Fernandez, 2021).

Now, when it comes to applying these stretching techniques, it is important to consider your workout's demands. For strength-focused workouts, you might find dynamic stretching during the warm-up and static stretching in the cool-down most beneficial. In contrast, endurance athletes may benefit from a combination of dynamic and PNF stretching to enhance flexibility and performance without compromising muscle stamina.

It is also worthwhile to integrate myofascial release regularly. This not only aids in recovery on rest days but enhances flexibility and can prevent injury. Given the stress repeated movements can place on the body, regular myofascial release can be a game-changer, particularly for those engaged in high-intensity training or those who are older and dealing with the natural stiffening of joints and tissues.

What about those recovering from injuries? PNF and myofascial release can be particularly useful. These methods help maintain muscle and fascia health without putting excessive strain on injuries. However, consultation with a professional is key to ensuring that stretching aids rather than hinders recovery.

For the military, athletes, and bodybuilders who engage in rigorous training regimes, incorporating a variety of stretching techniques tailored to their specific needs and recovery periods can significantly impact performance. Knowing when to apply each method, such as dynamic stretches before a drill or static stretches after a heavy lifting session, can make all the difference.

Now, let us talk about integrating these stretching methods into your routine efficiently. It is not merely about stretching; it is about stretching correctly and at the right time. Begin with dynamic stretches pre-workout to prepare your body. Post-workout, switch to static stretches to aid in recovery. Sprinkle in PNF and myofascial release as needed, particularly after workouts or on recovery days, to enhance flexibility and muscle health.

Remember, adaptability is key. Your body's needs can change based on a multitude of factors: the intensity of your workout, recovery phase, even the time of day. Listening to your body and adjusting your stretching routine accordingly can help in maximizing performance and minimizing injury risk.

In conclusion, stretching is an integral part of any fitness routine, not just for injury prevention but for enhancing performance and flexibility. By understanding the different types of stretching and their appropriate applications, you can create a more effective and comprehensive workout routine. Whether you are warming up, cooling down, or focusing on recovery, there is a stretching technique that fits your needs. So go ahead, stretch the right way, and see the difference it makes in your training and overall well-being.

Importance of Warm-ups

Warm-ups are like the appetizer to your workout meal. They signal your body, saying, "Hey, we're about to take things up a notch, so let's get ready!" It is not just about physically gearing up for the exercise; it is about tuning your mind into the workout zone, reducing the risk of injuries, and optimizing your performance. This section dives into why incorporating a proper warm-up routine is non-negotiable in achieving fast, real fitness results safely and effectively.

First off, warm-ups increase body temperature, which enhances muscle flexibility. Cold muscles are akin to uncooked spaghetti - rigid and easily broken. But warm them up, and they become like cooked spaghetti - flexible and resilient (Smith, 2019). This increased flexibility reduces the risk of tears and strains during more intensive exercises.

Moreover, warm-up exercises prepare your cardiovascular system for the upcoming workout, gradually increasing heart rate and promoting blood flow to muscles. This cardiovascular prep minimizes the shock on your system when you shift from rest to high activity. It is also crucial for distributing the much-needed oxygen and nutrients to muscles, enabling them to perform longer and stronger (Johnson et al., 2020).

Another pivotal benefit is injury prevention. Warm-ups do not just prepare your body; they are a critical step in preventing acute and overuse injuries. By gradually increasing muscle temperature and flexibility, the likelihood of sprains, strains, and muscle tears is significantly reduced. Considering that injuries can set you back in your fitness goals, the importance of warm-ups cannot be overstated (Williams & Anderson, 2018).

In the realm of blood occlusion training, warm-ups take on an even more significant role. This training method, which involves restricting blood flow to muscles to increase strength and muscle size with low-load exercises, requires that muscles be well-prepared to handle the unique stresses this technique places on them. A thorough warm-up ensures that muscles are ready for the peculiarity of blood flow restriction, enhancing both safety and effectiveness (Scott, 2021).

Warm-ups also prime the nervous system. Think of it as flipping the switch from 'rest' to 'active' mode. This activation is critical for improving reaction times and coordination during your workout, allowing you to perform exercises more efficiently and safely.

For individuals recovering from an injury, warm-ups are even more critical. They help reintroduce the body to physical activity in a controlled and gradual way, ensuring that the healing process is not disrupted. For athletes, a well-structured warm-up can mean the difference between a stellar and mediocre performance. It prepares their bodies and minds for the rigors of their sporting activity, enhancing focus and overall performance (Hall, 2020).

It is also worth mentioning the psychological benefits of warm-ups. They provide a mental transition period that helps you focus on your workout, set goals for the session, and mentally prepare for the challenge ahead. This mental preparation can enhance motivation and improve training outcomes.

For the elderly and individuals with chronic conditions, warm-ups are indispensable. They help in gradually raising the heart rate and increasing muscle temperature, which is crucial for minimizing stress on the heart and preventing injuries. Given the higher risk of injuries in older adults, a proper warm-up becomes even more essential in keeping fitness activities safe and enjoyable.

Now, considering the importance of warm-ups, it is crucial to tailor them to your specific activities. The right warm-up exercises can vary significantly depending on whether you are about to engage in strength training, cardio, or sports activities. Customizing your warm-up to the day's workout will ensure that the muscles and movements most involved are properly prepared (Smith, 2019).

Interestingly, the benefits of warming up extend beyond immediate workout performance. Research indicates that consistent warm-up routines can improve overall flexibility, leading to better long-term fitness and reduced injury risk (Johnson et al., 2020).

With all these benefits, it is a no-brainer that skipping warm-ups is not worth the risk. Not only do warm-up exercises ready your body and mind for upcoming workouts, but they also play a vital role in preventing injuries and enhancing overall flexibility in the long term. This makes them an essential component of any fitness regimen.

In conclusion, warm-ups are not a mere preamble to the main workout; they are a critical component of a comprehensive fitness routine. By adequately preparing your body for exercise, enhancing performance, and reducing the risk of injury, warm-ups enable safer, more effective workouts. They are especially vital in specialized training methods like blood occlusion training, where the unique stresses on the muscles require careful preparation to ensure both safety and efficacy.

Embracing warm-ups as an indispensable part of your fitness journey can significantly impact your overall training results. By ensuring your body is appropriately primed for the stresses of your workout, you are setting the stage for a safer, more effective, and ultimately, more enjoyable fitness experience.

Incorporating Flexibility Exercises into Your Routine: Cool-down Techniques to Prevent Injury

After a robust discussion on the significance of warm-ups and the different types of stretching, it is essential we pivot to a component equally vital to your fitness journey—cool-downs. As you have learnt to prime your muscles for the workout ahead, the period immediately following your exercise regime deserves just as much attention to prevent injury and aid in recovery.

Cool-downs essentially help in gradually lowering your heart rate and relaxing your muscles, which can be critical after intense physical exertion. Think of it as telling your body, "Hey, the hard part's over. Let us ease back into our normal pace." This transition is crucial for preventing dizziness and muscle stiffness, allowing for a smoother recovery process.

Incorporating flexibility exercises into your cool-down routine is a scientifically proven method to reduce the risk of injury (Smith, 2019). These exercises enhance not only your flexibility but also your overall physical performance by improving your range of motion and reducing muscular tension. Let us dive into some effective cool-down techniques that include flexibility exercises to keep your muscles happy and injury-free.

First, start with gentle dynamic stretches. Unlike the more intense dynamic stretches you might do in a warm-up; these are performed at a slower pace. Think of movements like arm circles, leg swings, or torso twists. These help in gradually decreasing your heart rate while keeping the muscles engaged.

Transitioning from dynamic to static stretching is the next step. While your muscles are still warm, it is the perfect time to work on improving your flexibility. Focus on major muscle groups that were heavily used during your workout. If you are a runner, for instance, emphasize your quadriceps, hamstrings, and calves. Hold each stretch for 30 seconds to 2 minutes for optimal results. Keep in mind, holding the stretch longer yields better results. If you are new to stretching, start with 30 seconds and gradually progress to 2 minutes. If you feel any discomfort, you have pushed the stretch too far.

Breathing is another aspect that cannot be overlooked during your cool-down. Deep, controlled breathing helps in oxygenating your muscles and facilitating the removal of lactic acid, which accumulates during vigorous activity. Pair each stretch with a deep breath in and a slow breath out, sinking

deeper into the stretch with each exhale.

Incorporating yoga poses such as the child's

pose, cobra pose, or downward-facing dog can also

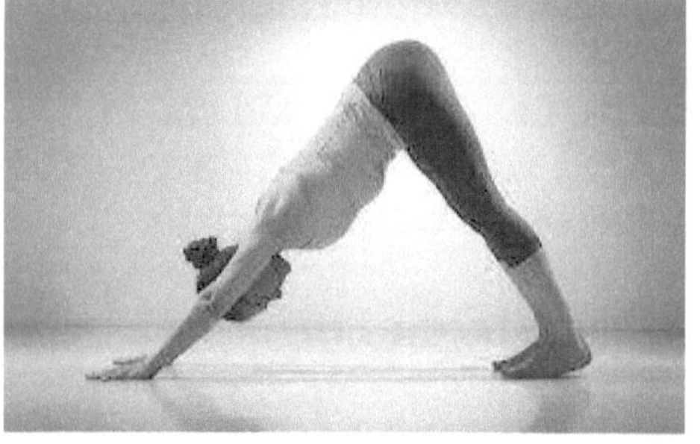 substantially benefit

your cool-down

routine. These poses

are excellent for

stretching multiple muscle groups at once and

promoting relaxation.

For those engaged in high-impact activities or

strength training, foam rolling can be an invaluable

addition to your cool-down routine. It is a form of self-

myofascial release that helps in alleviating muscle

tightness and improving blood flow. Spending a few

minutes rolling out your thighs, back, glutes, calves and

shoulders can make a significant difference in how you feel post-workout.

Mindfulness or meditation for a few minutes at the end of your cool-down can further enhance the relaxation and recovery process. This mental component aids in reducing stress and improving focus, rounding off the physical benefits perfectly.

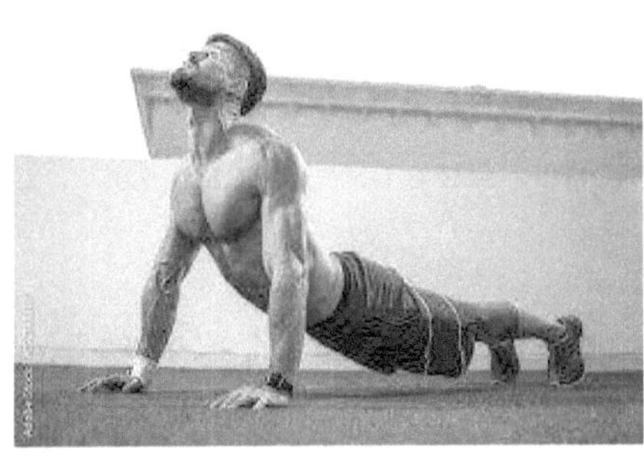

It is also worth noting that the flexibility exercises in your cool-down should be tailored to your specific needs and the intensity of your workout. What works for a bodybuilder might not be as effective for a marathon runner or someone recovering from an injury. Listening to your body and adjusting accordingly is key.

For individuals recovering from injuries, it is especially crucial to approach cool-downs cautiously. Depending on the nature of the injury, certain stretches or activities may need to be modified or avoided altogether. Consulting with a physical therapist or a fitness professional can provide personalized guidance.

Military personnel and athletes, whose physical demands can be exceedingly high, might find benefit in extending their cool-down period or incorporating additional recovery techniques, such as ice baths or compression garments, to aid in the process.

Similarly, the elderly or those new to exercise might prioritize gentle stretches and movements that focus on mobility and flexibility, in addition to emphasizing balance to prevent falls.

In conclusion, cool-downs are an indispensable part of any fitness regimen, with flexibility exercises playing a crucial role in preventing injuries and enhancing recovery. Remember, the goal is not just to get fit fast but to do so sustainably, keeping your body safe and injury-free. By integrating these techniques into your routine, you are not just cooling down; you are setting yourself up for continued success in your fitness journey.

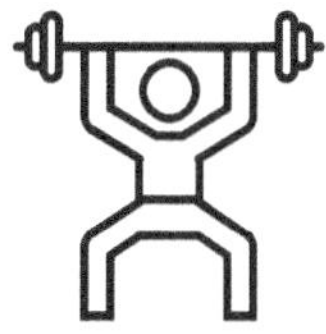

Chapter 6

Injury Prevention Strategies

We will now delve deeper into exploring strategies focused on injury prevention, extending beyond the basic warm-up and cool-down routines. Embarking on a fitness journey, whether you are an athlete, a fitness enthusiast, or someone navigating the recovery process, demands more than sheer willpower and discipline; it requires smart strategies to prevent injuries that could set you back. Injury prevention is not just about avoiding the pain and inconvenience associated with getting hurt. It is about understanding your body, knowing your limits, and using scientifically proven methods, like blood occlusion training, to achieve real results without overburdening your muscles and joints. This innovative approach not only maximizes your gains by tricking your body into thinking it is working harder than it actually is, but it also plays a crucial role in reducing the risk of injury. By applying the principles of blood flow restriction in a controlled manner, you create a safe, yet intensely effective workout environment. This chapter dives deep into various injury prevention strategies, elaborating on common exercise injuries and how to sidestep them, protective measures you can implement immediately, and the significance of rehabilitation and recovery. We will also delve into the critical balance of knowing when to push through and when to seek professional advice— a fundamental aspect of sustaining a long and fruitful fitness journey.

Understanding Common Exercise Injuries

When we talk about pushing our bodies to the limit, we are usually talking about our next level of fitness and strength. It is this drive that often sets us apart, but it is also a double-edged sword. Injuries are an almost inevitable part of any fitness journey but understanding them is the first step in preventing them. So, let us dive into the common injuries that can occur during exercise and how knowing about them can shape our training and recovery strategies.

First off, it is key to recognize that not all exercise injuries are due to bad form or pushing too hard. Sometimes, they are a result of overuse. This is when a specific muscle or joint has been worked repeatedly, to the point of stress, without adequate time for recovery. Think runner's knee or tennis elbow –

these are not just snazzy names; they are real issues that can sideline anyone from a beginner to a pro.

Then there is the acute injury, which happens in a blink of an eye. You are lifting heavier, running faster, and suddenly, you feel a snap or pop. This could be a sprained ankle, a pulled muscle, or even a tear in a tendon. Acute injuries are immediate and often unavoidable, striking without warning but usually during high-intensity activities.

Understanding injuries means also looking at why they occur. Besides overuse and acute incidents, improper form stands out as a major culprit. It is a silent threat; you might not even realize your form is off until it is too late. For instance, squatting with your knees buckled in can place undue stress on your joints, leading to pain and injury over time.

Ignoring pain is another pathway to injury. It is one thing to push through discomfort, but it is entirely another to ignore sharp or persisting pain. This kind of pain is your body's red flag, signaling that something is wrong and needs attention, whether it is a strained back or a stress fracture.

Skipping warm-ups and cool-downs is a mistake too often made. These are not just bookends to your workout; they are essential elements of injury prevention. A proper warm-up increases blood flow, making muscles more pliable and less prone to injury. Cool-downs, on the other hand, aid in recovery, gradually reducing heart rate and preventing stiffness.

But how do we prevent these injuries? Once we are familiar with the what and why, we can look at the how. Correcting form, listening to our bodies, and not skimping on warm-ups and cool-downs are a start.

Incorporating rest days into our routines is also crucial. Muscles need time to repair, and without that, the risk of injury escalates.

The role of equipment should not be overlooked either. Wearing the right shoes can prevent a multitude of foot and ankle injuries, just as using the correct weight and equipment for strength training can avoid unnecessary strain.

Then there is the approach of cross-training, which involves mixing up your workout routine to balance out muscle use and decrease the risk of overuse injuries. It is a way to keep your body guessing and prevent the repetitive stress of doing the same movements over and over.

Now, what about blood occlusion training, the crux of our fitness strategy? This technique involves restricting blood flow to muscles during low-intensity resistance training. It sounds counterintuitive, right? But hear me out. It is scientifically proven to result in muscle growth and strength gains without the need for heavy lifting. The great part? It is also shown promise in reducing the risk of common exercise injuries by promoting muscle growth under less strain (Loenneke et al., 2012).

So, where does that knowledge leave us? Knowing the potential injuries and understanding how they occur sets the foundation for preventing them. This does not mean we can avoid injuries entirely – no one can promise that – but it means we can reduce the risk and, should injuries occur, ensure a faster and safer recovery.

Let us also remember that personalizing our approach to fitness is key. Tailoring workouts, rest days, and recovery strategies to our individual needs and listening to our bodies will go a long way in keeping us healthy and active.

In conclusion, comprehending common exercise injuries is an essential part of our fitness journey. It helps us tweak our routines, avoid potential pitfalls, and embrace practices like blood occlusion training, which may offer a safer path to achieving our fitness goals. So, here is to training smarter, not necessarily harder, and keeping those common injuries at bay.

Preventive Measures to Reduce the Risk of Injury

Entering the realm of fitness, whether you are a seasoned athlete or someone just starting to dip their toes into the water, comes with its share of challenges, especially when it comes to steering clear of injuries. While pushing for faster real fitness results can be thrilling, it is crucial to remember that injury prevention is just as important, if not more so, for sustainable progress. This brings us to the importance of understanding and employing preventive measures to keep injuries at bay.

One of the most critical steps in injury prevention is familiarizing yourself with the concept of blood occlusion training. How could restricting blood flow possibly be beneficial? Yet, studies have shown that when applied correctly, this technique can enhance muscle strength and size, using much lighter weights than traditional strength training methods (Loenneke et al., 2012). This is not just good news for those who are short on time or do not have access to heavyweights; it is also a significant advancement in reducing the risk of injury.

Mindful movement is another cornerstone of injury prevention. It is easy to tune out while exercising, especially during repetitive activities. However, staying present and focused on your body's mechanics is essential. This means being aware of your posture, the alignment of your body, and making adjustments as needed to avoid placing undue strain on certain areas. For example, ensuring your knees maintain proper alignment behind your toes and keeping the weight on your heel during a squat can significantly reduce the risk of knee injuries.

Hydration plays a more substantial role in injury prevention than many realize. Dehydrated muscles and connective tissues become more susceptible to tears and strains. Therefore, ensuring you are adequately hydrated before, during, and after exercise is a simple yet effective way to reduce injury risk. The body's requirement can vary based on numerous factors but aiming for about 2 liters of water per day is a good baseline, with additional intake depending on the intensity and duration of your training (Popkin, D'Anci, & Rosenberg, 2010).

Another critical aspect of injury prevention is incorporating a well-rounded warm-up routine before diving into the main workout. This could include a combination of dynamic stretches and light cardio exercises to gradually increase your heart rate and blood flow to the muscles. By preparing your body for the more intense activity to come, you are less likely to suffer from strains and sprains.

Rest days are not an optional part of a training regimen; they are an integral component. Overtraining can quickly lead to burnout and injuries due to the cumulative stress it puts on the body. It is vital to listen to your body and give it the time it needs to recover. Integrating rest days into your routine allows your muscles to repair and strengthen, ultimately contributing to better performance and a reduced risk of injuries.

Nutrition cannot be overlooked when it comes to injury prevention. Consuming a balanced diet rich in vitamins and minerals supports muscle and bone health, aids in recovery, and reduces inflammation. Foods high in omega-3 fatty acids, calcium, and vitamin D should be staples in your diet to help fortify your body's defenses against the risk of injury.

The use of appropriate equipment also deserves attention. This includes footwear that provides the necessary support and shock absorption for your activities, as well as any protective gear relevant to your sport or training. Skimping on equipment can not only hinder your performance but also significantly increase the likelihood of an injury.

Dealing with early signs of discomfort promptly is key. Often, what starts as a minor niggle can escalate into a full-blown injury if ignored. Addressing symptoms early, whether through rest, modifying your training, or seeking professional advice, can prevent many common exercise-related injuries from worsening.

Adopting a balanced training regimen that includes both strength and flexibility workouts can markedly reduce the risk of injuries. Too often, the focus is placed solely on building muscle or endurance, neglecting flexibility. Yet, flexibility exercises enhance the range of motion and reduce the risk of muscle imbalances, both common causes of exercise-related injuries.

Avoiding sudden increases in training intensity or volume is also crucial. The body needs time to adapt to new stress levels. Incremental increases, often referred to as progressive overload, help ensure that you are challenging your body without overwhelming it.

Understanding the limits of your body is fundamental. While pushing your boundaries is part of progress, there is a fine line between this and risking injury by overstepping what your body is currently capable of handling. Developing this understanding takes time and often, a bit of trial and error, but it is crucial for long-term fitness success and injury prevention.

Lastly, education is one of the most powerful tools at your disposal. Understanding the proper techniques for your exercises and learning about your body's mechanics can dramatically reduce your injury risk. As with blood occlusion training, branching into new training methods should always be done with a solid foundation of knowledge and, when possible, under the supervision of a professional.

In conclusion, while the pursuit of fitness and strength is admirable, it is equally important to do so in a way that minds the well-being of your body. By implementing these preventive measures, you are not just safeguarding against injuries; you are laying the foundation for sustainable fitness progress that does not cut corners when it comes to your health.

Remember, it is about playing the long game, ensuring that every step taken towards achieving your fitness goals is a step taken with the well-being of your body in mind.

Rehabilitation and Recovery Techniques

Once an injury occurs, it is paramount to switch gears from prevention to effective rehabilitation and recovery. This transition is crucial, not only to mend the damage done but also to fortify the body against future injuries. It is where the science kicks in, and if you are savvy about it, recovery does not have to sideline you any longer than necessary.

One of the most advanced, yet underutilized, techniques in the world of recovery is blood occlusion training. This method, though sounding somewhat like something out of a sci-fi novel, is scientifically proven to speed up recovery, even from the comfort of your living room. As you learned in previous chapters, it involves restricting blood flow to the injured area to increase the concentration of growth hormones, which aids in rapid recovery (Loenneke et al., 2012).

But before you start tying tourniquets around your limbs, it is important to understand that proper technique is key. Blood occlusion training should be performed under guidance or after thorough research. The balance is delicate; too tight, and you risk further injury, too loose, and the technique will not be effective.

Parallel to using advanced recovery techniques like blood occlusion, the fundamentals of RICE (Rest, Ice, Compression, and Elevation) have not lost their charm. Incorporating RICE into your rehabilitation program offers a multipronged approach to recovery, combining the beneficial effects of blood occlusion with tried and tested injury management strategies.

Rehabilitation does not stop at physical techniques; nutrition plays an equally vital role. Feeding your body, the right nutrients can significantly impact your recovery speed. Protein is crucial for muscle repair, while vitamins and minerals from fruits and vegetables combat inflammation, supporting the body's healing mechanisms.

Hydration is another cornerstone of a successful recovery. Muscles are about 75% water and keeping 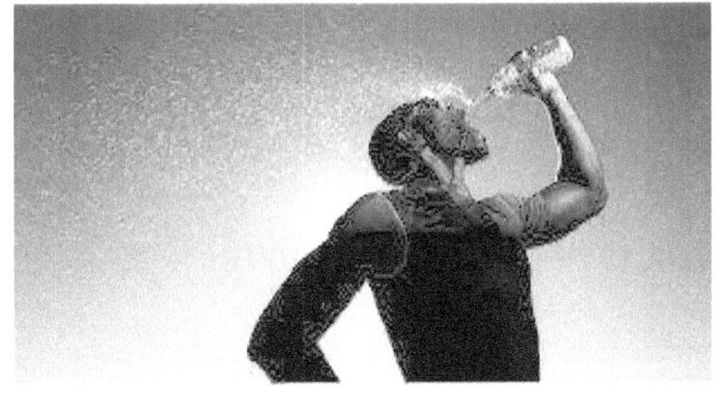 them hydrated is critical to prevent cramps and promote flexibility. Coupled with blood occlusion training or other physiotherapy techniques, staying well-hydrated ensures that your recovery is not hindered by preventable complications.

Movement, as paradoxical as it might seem, is also an essential component of rehabilitation. Early mobilization, within the pain-free limits, prevents the loss of muscle strength and joint stiffness. Techniques such as gentle stretching and mobility exercises can facilitate this process without imposing stress on the injured area.

The integration of mental health strategies into the recovery process cannot be overstated. Injuries can be frustrating, leading to feelings of isolation or depression. Mindfulness, meditation, and setting realistic goals for your rehabilitation can provide a more holistic recovery. This mental fortification complements the physical rehabilitation, making the process more bearable and even insightful.

In terms of protecting your body for future workouts, understanding the science of muscle building and recovery is beneficial. This knowledge allows for more informed decisions regarding workout plans, rest days, and when to push the limits. Education about the benefits of blood occlusion training and how it can be incorporated into a recovery plan is paramount for those looking to implement advanced techniques.

Consulting with professionals is another critical step in the recovery process. Whether it is a physical therapist for blood occlusion training guidance, a nutritionist for dietary advice, or a mental health professional for coping strategies, expert insight can tailor the recovery process to your specific needs, ensuring a safer and more effective rehabilitation.

Technological advancements have also brought about tools like compression sleeves that can be used for recovery. Furthermore, the traditional ice bath offers numerous scientifically proven benefits. They represent the bridge between traditional recovery methods and newer, scientifically backed techniques.

It is also essential to gradually reintroduce activity post-injury. Even after symptoms have subsided, the healed area may remain vulnerable for some time. A careful, methodical increase in activity allows the body to adapt without risking re-injury.

Preventative measures should be woven into the rehabilitation program to fortify against future injuries. Incorporating strength training, improving flexibility, and continuing to educate oneself on body mechanics can transform a recovery journey into an opportunity for overall physical improvement.

Lastly, patience is perhaps the most underestimated element in the recovery process. The desire to jump back into routine can be overwhelming but allowing the body the time it needs to fully recover is essential. Balancing the eagerness with a methodical and informed approach to rehabilitation ensures not only a complete recovery but a stronger comeback.

In conclusion, rehabilitation and recovery are multifaceted processes that require a careful balance of physical rehab techniques, nutritional support, hydration, mental health strategies, and, importantly, patience. By understanding and applying these principles in conjunction with innovative methods like blood occlusion training, individuals can achieve a more effective and efficient recovery, paving the way for a stronger, more resilient body ready to take on future challenges.

Knowing When to Rest and When to Seek Professional Help

In the journey of achieving peak fitness and pulling off those awe-inspiring physical feats, there's a less glamorous yet critical aspect we must discuss knowing when to hit the brakes and take a rest or, in more serious instances, seek professional help. This wisdom is crucial in the realm of injury prevention, especially when exploring avant-garde methods like blood occlusion training, a technique that is getting the nod for its efficiency in muscle building without the hefty weights.

Understanding the boundary between effective training stress and detrimental overreach is paramount. Train too lightly, and you are just going through the motions without real gains. Push too hard, and you might end up sidelined, nursing injuries instead of crushing your goals. But how do you recognize that fine line? The answer lies in tuning in to your body's signals and respecting its need for rest.

First off, it is essential to distinguish between general fatigue and the onset of a potential injury. General fatigue might manifest as muscle soreness or tiredness — common after a good workout. On the contrary, sharp, localized pain or discomfort that alters your movement patterns or capabilities signals a red flag. Ignoring such symptoms can escalate minor issues into major injuries, potentially throwing a wrench in your fitness journey.

Rest is not just a passive, do-nothing affair. It is an active component of training where recovery processes go into overdrive. This downtime allows muscle repair, adaptation, and growth, particularly when practicing blood occlusion training, which stresses muscles in a novel way. During rest periods, it is also a prime time to evaluate your training strategy and ensure it aligns with your body's responses. Rest days do not always have to be identical. On certain days, incorporating "active rest" activities like mobility exercises, stretching, or gentle cardio to boost circulation, improve range of motion and facilitate quicker recovery can be beneficial.

Now, let us get into the nitty-gritty of when to consider booking an appointment with a healthcare professional. If rest, coupled with basic home remedies like ice, compression, and elevation, does not alleviate pain or discomfort within a reasonable period — typically a few days — then checking in with a doctor is advisable. This is especially true for pain that persists during daily non-exercise activities.

Another scenario demanding professional attention is recurrent pain in the same area, even after taking ample rest. This could indicate a chronic issue or improper technique, something that professional intervention can diagnose and correct.

But it is not just about physical ailments. Feeling unusually fatigued, experiencing sleep disturbances, or a sudden drop in performance are potential indicators of overtraining syndrome, a condition entailing more than just physical exhaustion. Consulting with a health or fitness professional can provide insight into your condition, offering strategies for recovery and future prevention.

For individuals venturing into the realms of blood occlusion training, consulting professionals acquainted with this method beforehand can help tailor a program minimizing injury risk. Given the unique nature of this training, expert guidance ensures you are leveraging the technique effectively and safely.

Moreover, seeking professional help is not a sign of weakness or failure but a proactive approach to sustaining your fitness journey. It is about fine-tuning your regimen and embracing the fact that through recovery and professional guidance, you are setting the stage for greater achievements.

Remember, rest and recovery are not just about avoiding negatives like injury. They play a constructive role in your training regimen. Adequate rest boosts performance, aids in muscle development, and enhances overall well-being. It is the yin to the yang of active training within your blood occlusion training or any other fitness method for that matter.

It is also worth noting that preventive measures, like warm-up and cool-down techniques discussed in past sections, significantly contribute to knowing when to rest. These practices not only prepare your body for the strain to come but also facilitate recovery, lessening the likelihood of injury and the subsequent need for professional intervention.

In sum, embracing rest and recognizing when to seek professional help are not detours from your fitness goals but rather essential components of a sustainable, healthy fitness journey. By paying heed to your body's signals and erring on the side of caution, you are not just preventing injuries but also ensuring that your training remains effective, enjoyable, and lifelong. Your body will thank you for the mindfulness you bring to your training, ensuring not only rapid gains but also lifelong fitness and well-being.

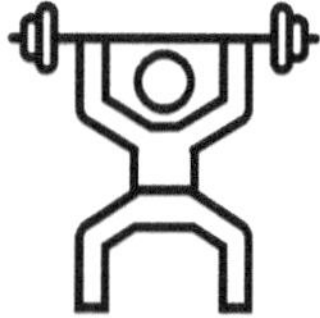

Chapter 7

Maximizing Nutrition for Accelerated Muscle Building: Athletes, Injured and Elderly

Shifting our focus from the gym to the kitchen, we will explore how nutrition is equally, if not more, vital for maximizing muscle growth and overall health and fitness. Combining blood occlusion training (BOT) with optimal nutrition and recovery strategies is crucial for maximizing muscle gains. Nutrition plays a transformative role by providing the building blocks for muscle repair and growth. Adequate protein intake, particularly the consumption of essential amino acids, is paramount for muscle synthesis, and this can be further optimized by ingesting protein shortly after a BOT session to take advantage of the anabolic window (Schoenfeld et al., 2017). Alongside protein, carbohydrates and healthy fats serve as vital energy sources, enabling you to perform at your peak during BOT. Carbohydrates can also mitigate muscle protein breakdown post-training, which supports the anabolic process. On the recovery front, rest and sleep are just as fundamental; during sleep, growth hormone levels elevate, facilitating muscle repair (Dattilo et al., 2011). Active recovery methods, such as low-intensity activities or stretching, may enhance circulation and nutrient delivery to the muscles, aiding in the repair process. Additionally, employing strategic hydration practices cannot be overstated, as even slight dehydration can impair performance and recovery (Popkin et al., 2010). By aligning your diet and recovery efforts with your BOT regimen, you are setting the stage for accelerated muscle building and improved overall fitness.

Navigating through the myriad of dieting approaches can feel like trekking through a labyrinth, but fear not, as this chapter sheds light on the top three dieting paradigms that have shown significant promise in optimizing nutrition. These are Intermittent Fasting, where timing is everything, Counting Macronutrients, which is akin to the financial budgeting of your food intake, and Carb Cycling, a strategic alteration of carbohydrate intake to fit your body's needs. Each approach has its unique framework and benefits, accommodating various lifestyles, fitness goals, and dietary needs. Particularly for the elderly, adhering to one of these approaches can be instrumental in maintaining muscle mass, bone density, and overall vitality. However, it is not just about choosing a diet; it is about integrating these nutritional strategies with an understanding of the body's changing needs as it ages. The emphasis here is on balance, ensuring adequate protein intake for muscle preservation (Houston et al., 2008), adjusting caloric intake as metabolic rates decline (Roberts, 2000), and ensuring sufficient vitamin D and calcium levels to support bone health (Boonen et al., 2006). This chapter is your guide not just to selecting a dieting approach that resonates with your life phase and fitness goals but also to maximizing your nutritional intake for longevity and quality of life, especially for our senior readers.

The Fuel for Muscle Mastery

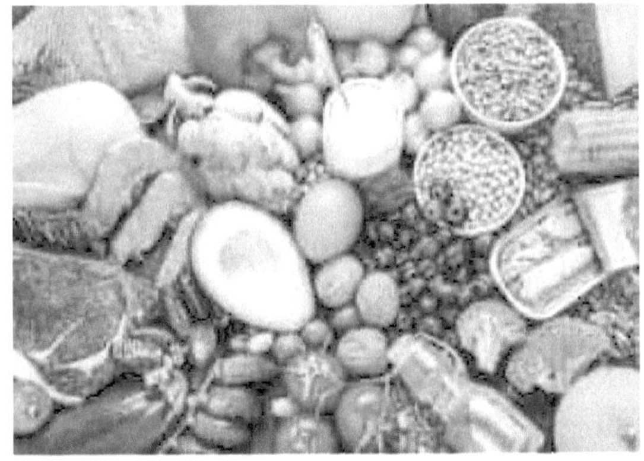

Nutrition is often overlooked in the quest for muscle growth, yet it plays a crucial role, especially when incorporating techniques like blood occlusion training (BOT). To understand the concept of feeding your muscles for mastery, it is imperative to grasp the symbiotic relationship between nourishment and optimized muscle function.

Proteins are the building blocks of muscle. To facilitate muscle repair and growth, a consistent intake of high-quality protein is central (Phillips & Van Loon,

2011). When engaged in BOT, where the stress on muscles is significant despite lower weights, ample protein becomes even more essential for recovery and growth. The recommendations from both the ISSN and ACSM advise an intake of approximately 1 gram of protein per pound of body weight for strength-training athletes (Prisk, 2020).

Proteins play a fundamental role in the body, serving as the building blocks of tissues, muscles, enzymes, hormones, and other essential molecules. They are composed of amino acids, which are crucial for various physiological processes and are categorized as either complete or incomplete based on their amino acid composition. Complete proteins contain all nine essential amino acids that the body cannot produce on its own and must be obtained from the diet. Sources of complete proteins include animal-based foods such as meat, poultry, fish, eggs, and dairy products. These proteins are considered high-quality proteins as they provide all the essential amino acids in adequate proportions, supporting optimal muscle growth, muscle repair, and maintenance of body tissues.

On the other hand, incomplete proteins lack one or more essential amino acids and are typically found in plant-based foods such as grains, legumes, nuts, seeds, and vegetables. While incomplete proteins may not provide all essential amino acids individually, they can be combined to form complementary protein sources that together provide a complete amino acid profile. For example, combining grains (e.g., rice, wheat) with legumes (e.g., beans, lentils) forms a complementary protein source that provides all essential amino acids (Nikholas, 2023). While some plant-based proteins may be lower in certain essential amino acids compared to animal-based proteins, a well-balanced vegetarian or vegan diet that includes a variety of plant-based protein sources can still meet protein requirements and support overall health.

In addition to providing amino acids for tissue repair and growth, proteins play a vital role in immune function, enzyme activity, hormone regulation, and fluid balance. They also serve as a source of energy, particularly during times of inadequate carbohydrate and fat intake or increased energy needs. Meeting protein requirements through a balanced diet that includes both complete and incomplete protein sources is essential for supporting optimal health and well-being at every stage of life. Whether obtained from animal or plant-based sources, prioritizing protein-rich foods as part of a balanced diet can help ensure adequate intake of essential amino acids and support overall health and vitality.

Carbohydrates cannot be ignored either; they are the primary source of energy for high-intensity training. Carbs help replenish glycogen stores that are depleted during workouts, thereby preventing muscle fatigue and aiding in the recovery process. Even though BOT does not use high-intensity exercise, carbohydrates are still important during any workout to provide energy. Some fast-digesting carbohydrates to provide energy during a workout would be bananas, white rice, apples, and sweet potato. According to the American College of Sports Medicine, it is recommended to consume 2.7 to 4.5 grams of carbohydrates per pound of body weight daily (Prisk, 2020).

Healthy fats have their place in the muscle mastery diet too. They are vital for hormone regulation, including testosterone, which plays a pivotal role in muscle synthesis. Healthy fats from sources like avocados, nuts, and fish contribute to an anabolic environment conducive to muscle growth.

Hydration is a key component that ties into nutrition. Water facilitates the transport of nutrients to muscles and assists in waste removal. Even mild dehydration can impair performance and recovery, making it a critical focus point. To calculate how much water a person should drink in one day, cut the body weight in half and drink that amount in ounces. (Cheuvront & Kenefick, 2014).

Micronutrients—vitamins and minerals—while required in smaller quantities, are essential for myriad functions, including energy metabolism and the synthesis of new muscle tissue. A BOT regimen demands seamless muscle function, which is supported by micronutrients.

Timing your meals is another nuanced aspect of nutrition for BOT practitioners. Ingesting protein and carbs post-workout can enhance muscle protein synthesis and replenish depleted energy stores, further supporting the benefits of occlusion training.

Specific amino acids like leucine have been highlighted for their role in triggering muscle protein synthesis. A diet or supplementation that ensures adequate leucine intake can serve to amplify the muscle-building signal post-BOT sessions, such as, lentils, beef, chicken, eggs, and salmon (Norton & Wilson, 2009).

Moreover, the role of creatine supplementation in supporting training cannot be overstated. Not only does it boost power and performance, but it also accelerates recovery between sets—ideal for BOT routines which rely on sustained performance over multiple rounds. Creatine is found in meat and fish products. However, creatine can be bought in supplement form for vegetarians. (Kreider et al., 2017).

Anti-inflammatory foods can contribute significantly to the recovery process. Elements such as omega-3 fatty acids found in fish oil help combat the inflammation induced by intense training, thereby aiding recovery and enabling consistent progress.

For individuals facing dietary restrictions or unique nutritional needs, tailor-fitting their BOT diet plan is a necessity. Whether it is due to personal ethics, intolerances, or a need for calorie control, understanding how to compile a nutritionally complete diet adaptable to BOT requirements is essential.

Meal planning and prep is a strategic step for ensuring your diet aligns with your BOT goals. Preparing meals in advance that meet the nutritional benchmarks for protein, carbs, fats, and micronutrients can mitigate the temptation of unhealthy snacks and keep you on track.

Adjusting your intake based on activity level is also a keen strategy. On days when you are engaged in BOT, upping your carb and protein intake can support the increased demands. Conversely, on rest days, a slight reduction, particularly in calorie-dense carbohydrates, can align with the reduced energy expenditure.

The holistic nature of nutrition in fostering muscle strength and recovery cannot be compartmentalized. It is a complex tapestry of macronutrients, micronutrients, hydration, timing, and even psychological satisfaction from enjoying your meals. All these aspects contribute to the foundational support necessary for BOT's unique stressors on the muscle groups and help maintain long-term success to reach your fitness goals.

With this comprehensive understanding of fueling for muscle mastery, individuals can adopt a nutrition regimen that complements their BOT routines, ultimately enhancing their performance, expediting recovery, and achieving accelerated muscle growth. Next, let us explore several well-known diets for muscle building: intermittent fasting, macronutrient tracking, and carb cycling. Each approach offers unique benefits tailored to specific

fitness goals.

Intermittent Fasting

Intermittent fasting (IF) has carved a significant niche in the world of health and fitness, gaining popularity for its versatility and potential health benefits. Contrary to the traditional dieting paradigm that focuses on what to eat IF centers around when to eat. It is not just about restricting calories; it is about cycling between periods of eating and fasting. This approach can make a profound impact on body composition and overall health, particularly when it is combined with smart eating during the eating windows.

At its core, IF can be tailored to fit various lifestyles and preferences, making it an attractive option for a wide audience—including the elderly, athletes, and those rehabilitating from injuries. The flexibility of IF lies in its different protocols, such as the 16/8 method, where you fast for 16 hours and eat during an 8-hour window, or the 24-hour fast, done once or twice a week.

Scientifically speaking, IF's benefits are rooted in the concept of metabolic switching—the body's transition from using glucose as its primary energy source to using fatty acids and their derivatives, ketones. This switch, which occurs during prolonged fasting periods, is thought to promote fat loss, improve metabolic health, and possibly extend lifespan (Mattson et al., 2017).

Furthermore, some studies also suggest that intermittent fasting may promote autophagy, a process by which cells remove damaged components and regenerate new ones, which could have anti-aging effects and protect against age-related diseases.

For the elderly population, IF presents a unique set of benefits and considerations. Age-related changes in metabolism and body composition, such as sarcopenia (the loss of muscle mass), can be mitigated through the careful application of IF, combined with adequate nutritional intake during eating periods. There's growing evidence suggesting that IF can enhance insulin sensitivity, reduce inflammation, and improve risk factors for chronic diseases such as heart disease and type 2 diabetes, all of which are crucial for the aging population (Ravussin & Redman, 2016).

For athletes and those engaged in intense physical training, IF can be strategically used to optimize body composition and performance. However, it is important to time fasting and feeding periods to support workout schedules. Ensuring nutrient-dense food intake during eating windows can help maintain energy levels, muscle recovery, and growth. Furthermore, the enhanced fat oxidation seen during fasting periods can benefit endurance athletes by improving their body's ability to utilize fat as a fuel source.

Post-injury, the recovery phase is critical, and nutrition plays a decisive role in it. IF, with its anti-inflammatory effects, may accelerate the healing process. Nonetheless, it is vital to ensure that during feeding windows, the focus is on foods rich in proteins, vitamins, and minerals to support tissue repair and recovery.

Implementing IF requires an understanding of one's own body and goals. Start with one of the less stringent fasting methods to see how your body responds. It is also beneficial to keep a journal to track progress and how you feel during fasting and eating windows.

Staying hydrated is essential during fasting periods. Water, black coffee, and tea are generally considered acceptable to consume while fasting, as they do not break the fast. However, avoid any beverages that contain calories.

One common concern about IF is the potential for overeating during feeding periods. It is crucial to focus on nutrient-dense foods and listen to the body's hunger cues to avoid this trap. Quality over quantity should be the mantra when it comes to choosing what to eat.

Another aspect to consider is social and family life. IF schedules can sometimes disrupt social eating patterns. It is essential to be flexible and adjust fasting periods when necessary to maintain a balance between social interactions and health goals.

For those looking to maximize fat loss, combining IF with exercise can accelerate results. The timing of workouts during the feeding window can enhance muscle synthesis and recovery. On the other hand, exercising during the fasting state can increase fat oxidation. However, it is crucial to listen to the body and adjust based on energy levels and overall well-being.

It is worth noting that IF is not suitable for everyone. Individuals with certain health conditions, such as diabetes, or those who are pregnant or breastfeeding, as it could impact maternal and fetal health, should consult with a healthcare provider before starting IF. Moreover, anyone who experiences negative side effects, such as extreme fatigue, irritability, or unwanted weight loss, should reconsider their fasting protocol.

In conclusion, IF offers a flexible approach to dieting that can benefit a wide range of individuals, including the elderly, athletes, and those recovering from injuries. By focusing on when to eat rather than just what to eat, IF can help improve metabolic health, body composition, and potentially increase lifespan. However, like any dietary approach, it should be tailored to individual needs and goals, with an emphasis on nutrient-dense foods during eating periods.

Remember, the key to successful dieting is sustainability. IF should not feel like a punishment but rather a lifestyle change that can bring about numerous health benefits. With the proper guidance and a mindful approach, intermittent fasting can be a valuable tool in achieving and maintaining optimal health.

Counting Macronutrients (Macros)

While exploring various dieting approaches, let us deep dive into the heart of one method that has been making waves among fitness enthusiasts, athletes, and even those simply looking to lead a healthier lifestyle. We are talking about counting macronutrients, also affectionately known as 'counting macros'. What is it about meticulously tracking our protein, fats, and carbohydrates intake that has everyone from bodybuilders to the elderly seeing impressive results? Let us unpack this, shall we?

First off, understanding what macros are is crucial. Macros, short for macronutrients, encompass the three nutrient types your body uses most: proteins, fats, and carbs. Proteins repair and build tissues, fats provide long-term energy, and carbohydrates fuel your day-to-day activities. For a well-rounded diet, you need a balance of all three, but the exact ratio can vary based on your fitness goals, age, and overall health.

Counting macros is not about restricting your diet to bland, unseasoned chicken breasts and broccoli. Instead, it is about hitting specific nutritional targets. It introduces a level of flexibility that is not commonly found in many diet plans. For example, if you are looking to build muscle, you might increase your

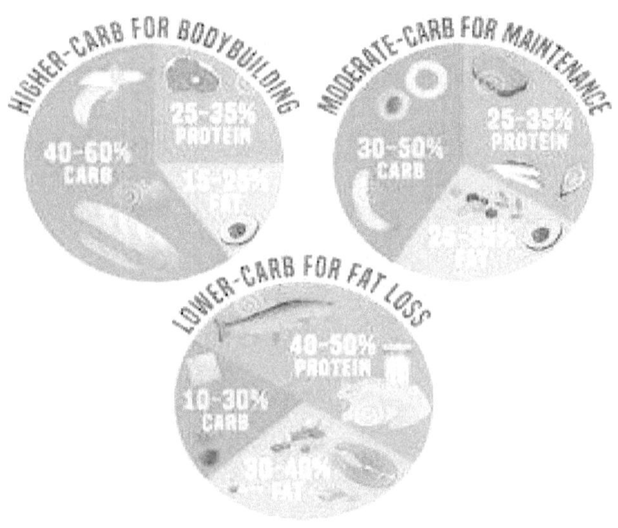

protein and carb intake. On the flip side, weight loss might require a higher protein but lower carb intake to preserve muscle mass while shedding fat.

The science backing this approach is solid. By tailoring your diet to your body's needs, you create an environment conducive to achieving your goals. Research has shown that diets focusing on macronutrient composition can influence body composition changes (Smith et al., 2014). This method empowers individuals by providing the knowledge and tools needed to make informed decisions about their food intake, emphasizing the quality of the nutrients consumed.

For the military members, athletes, and others in physically demanding professions, counting macros can optimize performance and recovery. An adequate intake of proteins and carbs can help in muscle recovery and energy replenishment after rigorous physical activities. This methodical approach ensures you are fueling your body adequately for both recovery and the energy demands of your next workout.

And what about our seniors? Nutritional needs change as we age, and a more meticulous approach to diet can support better health outcomes. Adjusting macronutrient intake can help manage or prevent chronic diseases commonly associated with aging, such as heart disease and diabetes. A focus on quality protein can aid in preserving muscle mass, which tends to decrease with age (Robinson et al., 2018).

So, how does one start counting macros? It begins with understanding your nutritional needs, which can be calculated based on factors like age, gender, weight, height, and activity level. Numerous online calculators can help you determine your daily macronutrient targets. Simply search for "Macronutrient calculator" on Google. Once you know your numbers, the next step is tracking your food intake, which can be done through a variety of free apps, such as, "my fitness pal" or use a good ol' fashioned food diary.

It is not just about numbers, though. Quality matters. Opting for whole, nutrient-dense foods will not only help you meet your macro targets but also fill your diet with vitamins, minerals, and fiber. This choice benefits overall health and not just your physique or performance.

Challenges do exist with counting macros. It requires discipline and a willingness to measure and record your food intake. Eating out or enjoying meals prepared by others can introduce inaccuracies. However, it is about progression, not perfection.

Making informed estimates in such situations can help you stay on track without becoming obsessive.

A common misconception is that counting macros is overly restrictive. On the contrary, it offers a liberating perspective on dieting. You can enjoy a wide variety of foods as long as you stay within your macro targets. While it is possible to include pizza and beer in your macronutrient goals, it is not advisable. This flexibility can make it easier to stick with over the long term, compared to diets that cut out entire food groups.

For those recovering from injuries, macro counting can be particularly beneficial. Tailoring your diet can help manage inflammation and support repair processes. A higher intake of protein, coupled with adequate fats and carbs, ensures your body has the necessary building blocks to recover, while the controlled caloric intake prevents unwanted weight gain during periods of reduced activity.

Wrapping up, counting macros is more than a diet trend; it is a science-based approach that offers flexibility, precision, and control over your nutrition. Whether you are a fitness rookie, a seasoned athlete, or someone navigating the nutritional needs of aging, mastering macro counting can be a game-changer. It is not just about looking good; it is about feeling good and making every calorie count towards your overall well-being.

Remember, the key is to find balance and enjoy the process. Nutrition is a vast and varied field, and what works for one person may not work for another. Tailoring your approach to fit your lifestyle, preferences, and goals is paramount. Taking the time to understand and implement macro counting can be a profound step towards achieving your health and fitness objectives.

So, whether you are looking to enhance your performance, recover from an injury, or simply lead a healthier life, give counting macros a shot. With a bit of practice, it can become second nature and possibly the best decision you make for your health.

Carb Cycling

Navigating the complex world of dieting can seem like an endless maze of do's and don'ts, especially when you are aiming for optimal nutrition and fitness gains. Among various dietary strategies, carb cycling stands out for its flexibility and effectiveness—a strategy that leverages the body's metabolic dynamics. In essence, carb cycling involves alternating between high-carb and low-carb days to fuel exercise performance while fostering fat loss and muscle growth. Carb cycling helps to keep your metabolism active, preventing it from slowing down and ensuring continuous fat burning.

The fundamental premise of carb cycling is it syncs your carbohydrate intake with your energy needs, varying the amount depending on the intensity of your exercise on a given day. On heavy workout days, a high carb intake fuels your muscles, enhancing your performance and aiding in recovery. Conversely, on rest or low-intensity days, reducing carb intake can help manage insulin levels and encourage fat burning. This strategic modulation can offer a dual advantage: it supports muscle growth while helping shed unwanted fat, aligning with the fitness goals of many athletes, military personnel, bodybuilders, and even those in recovery from injuries.

For elderly individuals, the approach might need a slight tweak. Aging bodies have different metabolic and nutritional needs. A moderate version of carb cycling can aid in maintaining muscle mass, which tends to diminish with age, while also managing weight and blood sugar levels. The key is to ensure a balanced intake of nutrients, prioritizing whole, unprocessed foods rich in fiber on lower carb days to sustain energy and overall health.

Scientific evidence underpinning carb cycling, though still emerging, is promising. Research indicates that altering carbohydrate intake can impact body composition, aiding in reducing fat mass while preserving or increasing lean body mass (Smith, 2014). Thus, for those engaged in fitness routines or looking to optimize their physique—especially without spending excessive hours in the gym—carb cycling can be a powerful tool.

Implementing carb cycling into your diet demands an understanding of your body's energy requirements and a meticulous plan. It is crucial to factor in your exercise intensity, duration, and goals. High-carb days should coincide with your most intense workouts, such as Blood Occlusion Training or long-duration cardio sessions. These high-carb days might include oats, rice, pasta, and potatoes in larger quantities, providing the fuel your body needs.

Conversely, low-carb days focus on lean proteins, healthy fats, and vegetables, reducing reliance on carbohydrates to encourage the body to burn fat for energy. Foods like chicken breast, avocado, nuts, and green leafy vegetables become staples, ensuring you still receive essential nutrients while cutting carbs.

One common concern with carb cycling is the potential complexity. However, with some initial planning and a bit of habit-forming, it becomes an intuitive approach to eating. Keeping a food diary, using nutrition tracking apps, or planning meals ahead can minimize decision fatigue and ensure adherence to the cycling pattern.

Hydration is another critical component, especially on high-carb days when the body tends to retain more water. Ensuring adequate fluid intake is essential to support metabolic processes and aid in recovery and performance.

Still, it is important to remember that individual responses to different macronutrient distributions can vary. Some may find they thrive with higher or lower carbohydrate intakes, even on designated days. Listening to your body's feedback and adjusting accordingly is crucial. Consulting with a nutritionist or dietitian can provide personalized guidance to tailor the approach based on your unique needs and health status.

For those new to carb cycling, starting slowly can help ease the transition. Begin by introducing a single high-carb day into your week, aligned with your most strenuous workout day. As you become more comfortable and observe how your body responds, additional high-carb days can be incorporated progressively.

It is important to not overlook the psychological benefits of carb cycling. This dietary strategy can alleviate the mental strain associated with more restrictive diets. By allowing flexibility and periodic indulgence in higher-carb foods, it can help maintain motivation and adherence over the long term. The built-in variety ensures that the diet never feels monotonous, potentially boosting overall satisfaction and sustainability.

Finally, carb cycling is not a one-size-fits-all solution. It is paramount to consider individual metabolic health, activity levels, and dietary preferences. For some, the benefits in terms of improved body composition and performance will be significant, making it a worthwhile approach to nutrition and fitness optimization.

Understanding and navigating the nuances of carb cycling can empower individuals across a spectrum of fitness levels and life stages to achieve their health and performance goals. By strategically modulating carbohydrate intake, you can support your body's needs for both exercise fuel and recovery, all while promoting a leaner body composition.

Nutritional Strategies for Healthy Aging

Nutrition plays a vital role in maintaining health and well-being, especially as we age. For the elderly, it becomes even more crucial to ensure proper nutrition to support overall health, immune function, and quality of life. As metabolism slows down and energy needs decrease with age, it is essential to focus on nutrient-dense foods that provide essential vitamins, minerals, protein, and fiber while limiting empty calories from added sugars and unhealthy fats.

A balanced diet for the elderly should include a variety of nutrient-rich foods such as fruits, vegetables, whole grains, lean proteins, and healthy fats. Fruits and vegetables are rich in vitamins, minerals, and antioxidants that help protect against chronic diseases and support immune function (Alhazmi, A et al., 2023).

Whole grains provide fiber for digestive health and slow-release carbohydrates for sustained energy levels. Lean proteins like poultry, fish, beans, and legumes are essential for muscle maintenance, repair, and immune function, especially in the elderly who may be at risk of muscle loss. Healthy fats from sources like nuts, seeds, avocados, and olive oil provide essential fatty acids that support heart health and cognitive function.

Iron and calcium are essential nutrients for elderly individuals, playing crucial roles in maintaining overall health and well-being. Iron is necessary for the production of hemoglobin, the protein in red blood cells that carries oxygen from the lungs to the rest of the body. Inadequate iron intake can lead to iron deficiency anemia, characterized by fatigue, weakness, and impaired immune function. For elderly individuals, iron deficiency anemia can be a common concern due to factors such as decreased absorption of iron from the diet and blood loss from gastrointestinal issues. Therefore, it is important for the elderly to consume iron-rich foods such as lean meats, poultry, fish, beans, lentils, and fortified cereals to maintain optimal iron levels, increase energy and prevent anemia (Chen, J et al., 2022)

Calcium is another critical nutrient for the elderly, essential for maintaining strong and healthy bones and teeth. As we age, bone density tends to decrease, increasing the risk of osteoporosis and fractures. Adequate calcium intake, along with vitamin D and weight-bearing exercise, can help slow down bone loss and reduce the risk of fractures. Dairy products such as milk, yogurt, and cheese are excellent sources of calcium, but for those who are lactose intolerant or have dairy allergies, calcium-fortified foods and beverages, leafy green vegetables, tofu, almonds, and sardines with bones are alternative sources. Additionally, calcium supplements may be recommended for elderly individuals who are unable to meet their calcium needs through diet alone. Ensuring adequate intake of both iron and calcium is crucial for promoting optimal health and well-being in the elderly population, supporting overall vitality and quality of life.

In addition to nutrient-rich foods, hydration is also crucial for elderly individuals, as dehydration can lead to a range of health issues such as urinary tract infections, constipation, and confusion. Encouraging regular fluid intake, including water, herbal teas, and broth-based soups, is important to prevent dehydration and maintain proper hydration levels.

Moreover, it is essential to address any specific dietary concerns or medical conditions that may affect nutrient absorption or metabolism in the elderly, such as diabetes, high blood pressure, or gastrointestinal issues. Consulting with a registered dietitian or healthcare professional can help tailor a nutrition plan that meets individual needs and promotes optimal health and well-being in the elderly population.

The Healing Diet for Injuries

When dealing with a musculoskeletal injury, proper nutrition becomes crucial for supporting the body's healing process and minimizing inflammation. A diet rich in nutrients that promote tissue repair, reduce inflammation, and support overall health can play a significant role in recovery. One key component of such a diet is ensuring an adequate intake of protein, which is essential for repairing damaged tissues and promoting muscle recovery. Lean protein sources such as poultry, fish, beans, lentils, tofu, and low-fat dairy products can help meet increased protein needs during the healing process.

In addition to protein, it is important to prioritize foods that are rich in anti-inflammatory nutrients, such as omega-3 fatty acids, antioxidants, and vitamins and minerals like vitamin C, vitamin E, and zinc. Omega-3 fatty acids, found in fatty fish like salmon, mackerel, and sardines, as well as walnuts, flaxseeds, and chia seeds, have been shown to have anti-inflammatory properties and may help reduce inflammation associated with musculoskeletal injuries. Similarly, antioxidant-rich foods like berries, leafy greens, nuts, and seeds can help combat oxidative stress and support tissue repair (Mendonça et al., 2020).

Furthermore, maintaining a balanced diet that includes a variety of fruits, vegetables, whole grains, and healthy fats can provide essential nutrients needed for overall health and well-being. Foods rich in vitamin C, such as citrus fruits, strawberries, bell peppers, and broccoli, can support collagen production and connective tissue repair. Incorporating foods high in vitamin E, such as almonds, sunflower seeds, spinach, and avocado, can help protect cell membranes from damage and promote tissue healing. Additionally, foods rich in zinc, such as lean meats, seafood, nuts, seeds, and whole grains, play a role in immune function and wound healing (Mendonça et al., 2020).

While proper nutrition is essential for supporting recovery from musculoskeletal injuries, it is also important to stay hydrated and maintain a healthy body weight to reduce excess stress on injured tissues. Drinking an adequate amount of water and avoiding excessive consumption of sugary or caffeinated beverages can help support hydration and overall health.

Working with a registered dietitian or healthcare professional can help tailor a nutrition plan that meets individual needs and supports optimal healing and recovery from musculoskeletal injuries. By prioritizing nutrient-dense foods, supporting tissue repair and reducing inflammation, and maintaining overall health and well-being, a well-balanced diet can play a critical role in the rehabilitation process for musculoskeletal injuries.

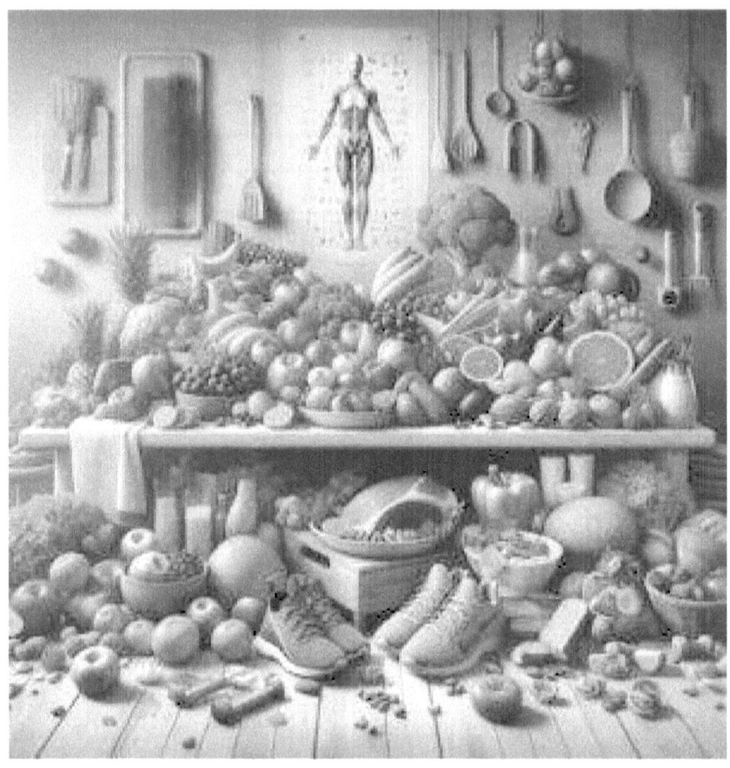

Going the Extra Mile

It is worth noting that among the various diet plans discussed earlier, there is an opportunity to elevate your nutrition to the next level and refine your diet even further. This can be achieved by incorporating the Paleo diet, in conjunction with the other diets discussed earlier. Since the Paleo diet focuses on 'what' you eat rather than 'how' you eat, you can incorporate this approach into any of the previously mentioned diets to significantly accelerate your fitness goals.

What is the Paleo diet? This diet, also known as the Paleolithic or caveman diet, is a dietary approach that seeks to mimic the eating habits of our ancient ancestors from the Paleolithic era. The fundamental principle of the Paleo diet is to consume foods that would have been available to our hunter-gatherer ancestors before the advent of agriculture and modern food processing techniques. This typically includes lean meats, fish, fruits, vegetables, nuts, and seeds, while excluding processed foods, grains, dairy, and refined sugars.

One of the key benefits proponents of the Paleo diet claim is its emphasis on whole, nutrient-dense foods. By focusing on fresh produce, lean proteins, and healthy fats, adherents often report feeling more satisfied and experiencing improved energy levels throughout the day. Additionally, since the diet eliminates processed foods and refined sugars, it can help regulate blood sugar levels and promote weight loss.

Moreover, the Paleo diet is often praised for its potential to reduce inflammation in the body. By excluding grains and legumes, which contain anti-nutrients such as lectins and phytates that can irritate the gut lining, some individuals find relief from digestive issues and autoimmune conditions. Additionally, the emphasis on omega-3-rich fish and grass-fed meats provides a good balance of essential fatty acids, which may further contribute to reducing inflammation and supporting overall health.

However, critics of the Paleo diet argue that it can be restrictive and may lead to deficiencies in certain nutrients if not properly planned. For example, the exclusion of grains and dairy products could result in inadequate intake of calcium, vitamin D, and B vitamins if alternative sources are not included in the diet. Additionally, some people may find it challenging to sustain the Paleo diet long-term, especially in social situations or when dining out.

In conclusion, the Paleo diet offers a whole-food approach to eating that prioritizes nutrient-dense foods and avoids processed ingredients. While it may have benefits such as improved energy levels, weight loss, and reduced inflammation for some individuals, it is essential to ensure a balanced intake of nutrients and consider individual preferences and lifestyle factors when adopting any new dietary approach. It is merely another approach to propel your fitness goals forward.

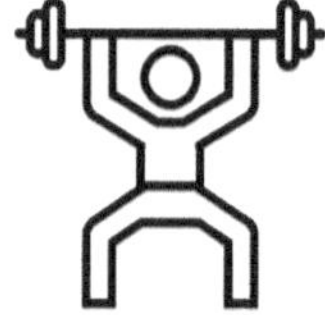

Chapter 8

Decoding Food Labels and Marketing Strategies, along with Meal Preparation and Cooking Pointers

Navigating the world of nutrition is not just about choosing the right types of food; it is equally important to understand what is actually in the food you are eating and how it's being marketed to you. Labels and marketing can often be misleading, with terms like "natural" and "organic" frequently thrown around without much regulation. Learning to decode these labels is crucial for making informed decisions that align with your fitness and health goals. For instance, understanding that a product labeled "trans fat-free" can still contain up to 0.5 grams of trans fat per serving can be a game-changer in maintaining a healthy diet (FDA, 2018).

Meanwhile, meal preparation is not just about cooking; it is a strategic approach to ensure you are fueling your body efficiently. It involves allocating time to prepare meals in advance, which can significantly enhance your diet's nutritional quality. This strategy can help athletes, bodybuilders, and fitness enthusiasts meet their rigorous nutritional requirements without resorting to less healthy, on-the-go options.

Plus, understanding cooking techniques can further optimize the nutritional value of your meals, making each calorie count even more. Whether you are looking to build muscle, lose weight, or simply maintain a healthy lifestyle, mastering these skills can have a profound impact. So, let us dive into the fine print of food labels and explore practical meal prep and cooking tips that can turn your kitchen into a powerhouse of nutrition.

Interpreting Nutrition Labels

Navigating the maze of nutrition labels can often feel like you are decoding a particularly tricky secret spy message. Yet, understanding these labels is essential, especially for anyone invested in fitness goals, be it athletes, military personnel, bodybuilders, or those recovering from injuries. Let us break down these labels into something a bit more digestible.

First off, the serving size is your key starting point. It is easy to overlook this part, but trust me, it is where a lot of us trip up. The amounts of calories, fats, carbohydrates, and proteins listed are all based on this serving size. So, if you eat double the serving size listed, remember you are also doubling all those numbers too.

Another marketing tactic to watch out for is the use of misleading serving sizes. Manufacturers often use smaller serving sizes to make their products appear lower in calories, sugar, or fat than they actually are. It is essential to pay attention to both the serving size and the number of servings per container to accurately assess the nutritional content of a product and avoid overconsumption.

Next up, calories. They are the big numbers that catch your eye, right? Calories are a measure of energy and keeping track of them is crucial whether you are looking to lose weight, gain muscle, or maintain your current fitness level. However, not all calories are created equal. It is where the type of nutrients making up those calories becomes critical.

Speaking of nutrients, let us chat about fats, carbs, and proteins - the major players on the nutrition label. Fats, both saturated and unsaturated, are necessary for a healthy diet but in moderation.

Carbohydrates include sugars and fibers, with a growing emphasis on the benefits of high-fiber foods for overall health and well-being. Proteins, a favorite among bodybuilders and anyone looking to build or repair muscle, are pivotal, and the label will tell you how much a single serving contributes to your daily requirements.

The % Daily Value (%DV) is another section you cannot ignore. These percentages help you understand how much a nutrient in a serving of food contributes to a daily diet, based on a 2,000 calorie-per-day diet. For anyone engaged in intense training or recovery, these values might need adjustments, but they offer a good baseline for comparison.

Ingredients lists are where food labels often reveal their true colors. Ingredients are listed in order of quantity, from highest to lowest. This can help you spot added sugars, unhealthy fats, and other additives you might want to avoid. Plus, for those with allergies or dietary restrictions, this part of the label is non-negotiable.

Look for products with simple ingredient lists containing recognizable, real-food ingredients and avoid those with long lists of artificial additives, preservatives, and refined sugars. Prioritize whole, minimally processed foods whenever possible. Additionally, aim to choose products that are high in fiber, protein, and essential nutrients and low in added sugars, unhealthy fats, and sodium.

But why does any of this matter? Knowing what goes into your body can significantly impact your fitness outcomes. For instance, a high-protein, low-sugar diet might support muscle recovery and growth, aligning perfectly with blood occlusion training methods that aim to maximize fitness gains without overburdening the body. Similarly, understanding nutrient timing and how different foods can support or hinder your fitness journey becomes clearer when you know what is on your plate.

Furthermore, with the rise of misleading marketing strategies, being able to cut through the noise and make informed choices about your diet is more important than ever. One common tactic is using terms like "low-fat," "sugar-free," or "all-natural" to imply that a product is healthy, even if it is high in other undesirable ingredients like added sugars, artificial sweeteners, or preservatives. Similarly, products labeled as "organic" or "gluten-free" may still be high in calories, unhealthy fats, or sodium, so it is crucial to look beyond these claims not just the flashy front packaging and examine the full ingredient list and nutrition facts panel. By becoming proficient in label reading, you empower yourself to make choices that align with your fitness and health goals.

In conclusion, interpreting nutrition labels is a skill that pays off in dividends. It is about more than just numbers; it is about understanding what your body needs to perform at its best, no matter your fitness level or goals. So next time you find yourself puzzled in the grocery aisle, take a moment to decode that label. Your body (and your fitness goals) will thank you.

Benefits of Meal Prepping

Focusing on the nutritional aspect of fitness, understanding the benefits of meal prepping becomes an essential component of your overall strategy. Meal prepping, in its essence, involves planning, preparing, and storing your meals in advance. It is a strategy that can significantly contribute to your fitness goals, whether you are an athlete, bodybuilder, or someone looking to enhance their physical condition through blood occlusion training. The advantages of meal prepping span various aspects, from time management to nutrition optimization, and understanding these benefits can elevate your fitness routine.

One of the primary benefits of meal prepping is the control it gives you over your diet. By planning your meals in advance, you can ensure that each meal is balanced and fits within your nutritional goals (Smith et al., 2019). This is especially beneficial when you are following specific diet approaches, like counting macros or intermittent fasting, as it allows you to accurately measure and distribute your intake of proteins, fats, and carbohydrates throughout the day.

Moreover, meal prepping can lead to significant time savings. By dedicating a few hours to prepare your meals, you free up time that would otherwise be spent cooking daily and reducing stress throughout the week. For those with busy schedules or intense training regimens, this can be a game-changer, giving you more time to focus on your fitness and recovery, and less time worrying about what your next meal will be.

Financial savings are another notable advantage. Buying ingredients in bulk and avoiding last-minute takeout or convenience food purchases can reduce your overall food expenditure. The initial effort of meal planning, and preparation pays off by minimizing waste and ensuring that every purchased ingredient is utilized effectively.

To meal prep effectively, start by planning your meals and snacks for the upcoming week, taking into account your nutritional needs, dietary preferences, and schedule. Choose recipes that are simple, balanced, and versatile, allowing you to prepare large batches of food that can be easily portioned out and enjoyed throughout the week.

Once you have selected your recipes, create a shopping list and gather all the necessary ingredients to streamline the meal prep process. Set aside a dedicated block of time, such as a few hours on the weekend, to batch cook and assemble your meals. Use this time to chop vegetables, cook proteins, prepare grains and starches, and portion out individual servings into storage containers. Investing in high-quality storage containers and labeling each meal with the date and contents can help keep your meal prep organized and ensure freshness.

When meal prepping, it is also important to consider cooking techniques that help retain the nutritional value of your food. Opt for cooking methods like steaming, boiling, baking, grilling, or sautéing with minimal oil to preserve the natural flavors and nutrients of your ingredients. Avoid deep-frying or overly processing foods, as these methods can strip away nutrients and add excess calories and unhealthy fats. Additionally, aim to include a variety of colorful fruits and vegetables in your meals to maximize nutrient intake and support overall health and well-being (Laustsen, 2023).

To further enhance nutrient retention, consider incorporating cooking techniques that help unlock the nutritional benefits of certain foods. For example, lightly cooking or blanching vegetables can help soften their cell walls, making nutrients more accessible for absorption. Similarly, soaking grains and legumes before cooking can reduce their phytic acid content, improving digestibility and nutrient absorption. Experiment with different cooking methods and techniques to find what works best for you and your dietary preferences, and do not be afraid to get creative in the kitchen!

For those engaging in blood occlusion training, nutrition plays a pivotal role in maximizing the training benefits. Meal prepping ensures that you have the right nutrients available to fuel your workouts and support recovery. The strategic timing of nutrient-dense meals can enhance muscle gain and recovery times, making it an indispensable tool for anyone following this training methodology.

Additionally, meal prepping helps in maintaining consistent portion sizes, which is crucial for weight management and body composition goals. Pre-portioned meals prevent overeating and can help maintain a caloric deficit or surplus, depending on your objectives, by providing just the right amount of food needed for each meal (Jones, 2020).

Meal prepping also encourages dietary variety, which is important for covering all micronutrient needs and preventing diet fatigue. By planning different meals for the week, you are more likely to include a wide range of vegetables, fruits, proteins, and grains, ensuring that your diet remains interesting and nutritionally balanced.

For individuals with specific dietary needs, such as athletes, the elderly, or those rehabilitating from injuries, meal prepping can ensure that dietary restrictions and requirements are met. Customizing meals to cater to specific health conditions or nutritional needs is easier when meals are planned and prepared in advance.

Lastly, meal prepping can be a powerful educational tool. By regularly engaging in the process of planning and preparing meals, individuals can learn more about nutrition, cooking techniques, and portion control. This knowledge not only aids in achieving fitness goals but also promotes long-term health and wellness.

In conclusion, the benefits of meal prepping are manifold and can significantly contribute to achieving fitness goals, supporting rigorous training regimens like blood occlusion training, and promoting overall health. By offering control over your diet, saving time and money, and ensuring that your nutritional needs are met, meal prepping is an invaluable strategy for anyone serious about their fitness and health.

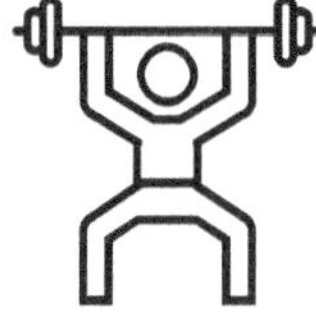

Overcoming Plateaus and Advancing Your Progress

Just when you think you have hit your stride in your fitness regimen and nutrition, you are blindsided by the dreaded plateau. But fear not; Chapter 9 unpacks the ins and outs of overcoming these hurdles and propelling your progress further with blood occlusion training (BOT). By cracking deep into the physiology of plateaus, we discover that the body's adaptation to stress is a natural occurrence (Smith et al., 2018). However, through strategic BOT application, including fine-tuning pressures and varying limb occlusion, we can reignite muscle growth and strength adaptations (Takarada et al., 2000). Additionally, this chapter guides you through identifying personal plateaus and tweaking your BOT protocol to shatter them—because progress is not linear, it is about knowing when and how to push the envelope. We will explore evidence-based strategies that highlight the importance of program variation and incremental intensification, ensuring that each workout continues to challenge your muscles and cardiovascular system, paving the way for continuous improvement and growth (Laurentino et al., 2012).

Strategies for Continued Growth

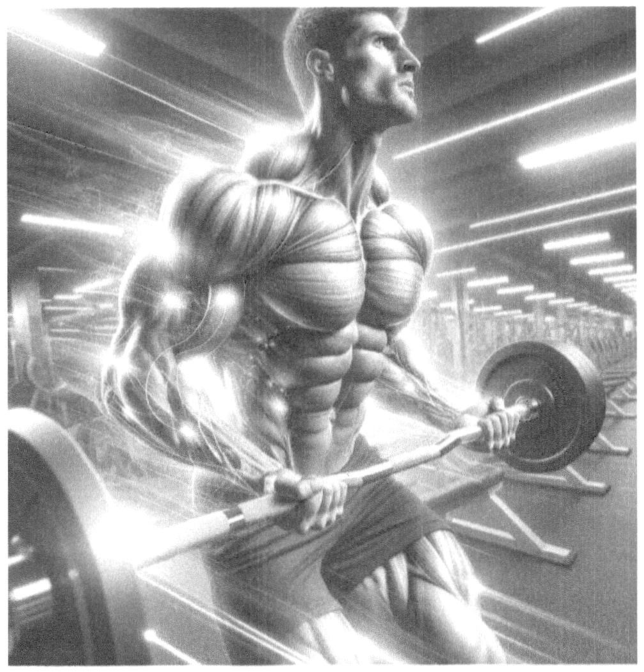

In the world of fitness, progress is often visualized as a linear path. But the reality for anyone dedicated to their physical development is that the journey is far more akin to the ebb and flow of tides. There are periods of rapid advancement and, inevitably, the frustrating plateaus where gains seem to be at a standstill. This is where strategies for continued growth become key, especially in the realm of blood occlusion training (BOT).

One critical aspect of continued growth is the reassessment of workout parameters. Progression does not mean increasing the occlusion band tightness, which is NEVER done. Always, stick to a 7 out of 10 tightness. Instead, it involves tweaking the factors that influence muscle adaptation. This means varying the time under tension, adjusting rest periods, and experimenting with different exercises and angles to continually challenge the muscles (Scott et al., 2015).

Another strategy is to integrate periodization into your BOT program. Periodization is the systematic planning of athletic or physical training. It involves progressive cycling of various aspects of a training program during a specific period. It is not only about changing the exercises but also manipulating the volume and intensity over time to optimize gains and reduce the risk of overtraining (Laurent et al., 2020).

The integration of supersets and drop sets within a BOT routine can also push past plateaus. These intensity techniques involve performing two exercises consecutively with minimal rest or reducing the weight without rest, respectively. Also, using BOT as a finisher set after each exercise would give that extra edge in your training. This approach can enhance muscle hypertrophy through increased metabolic stress—one of the drivers of growth facilitated by blood flow occlusion.

A **drop set** is a high-intensity weightlifting technique that involves performing a set of an exercise to failure, then immediately reducing the weight and continuing to perform more repetitions until reaching failure again (Johnson, 2023). This method is designed to push the muscles to fatigue and stimulate further muscle growth by recruiting different muscle fibers.

Benefits of drop sets include increased muscle hypertrophy, improved muscular endurance, and enhanced metabolic stress. However, it is essential to use drop sets judiciously as they can be highly demanding on the muscles and central nervous system. Incorporating drop sets into your workout routine can help break through plateaus and challenge your muscles in new ways for continued progress and growth. Always prioritize proper form and listen to your body's cues to prevent injury and optimize results.

A **superset** is a weightlifting technique where you perform two different opposing exercises back-to-back with little to no rest in between. For example:

back and chest, biceps and triceps, or quadriceps and hamstrings. Supersets are typically used to increase the intensity of a workout, improve muscular endurance, and save time by targeting different muscle groups in quick succession.

Benefits of supersets include increased workout efficiency, improved muscular endurance, and enhanced calorie burn due to the continuous movement between exercises. Additionally, supersets can help break through plateaus by challenging the muscles in new ways and promoting muscle growth. Incorporate supersets into your workout routine strategically, alternating between exercises that target different muscle groups to maximize results while minimizing fatigue. As with any exercise technique, prioritize proper form and listen to your body's cues to prevent injury and optimize performance.

A **finisher set** is a high-intensity exercise or series of exercises performed at the end of a workout to push muscles to fatigue and maximize metabolic stress (Lapidos & Lapidos, 2022). Finishers are commonly used to add an extra challenge, burn additional calories, and promote muscle growth.

Finisher sets offer several benefits that can enhance your workout routine. Firstly, they contribute to increased calorie burn by incorporating high-intensity exercises that elevate your heart rate and metabolic rate. This elevated metabolism can continue to burn calories even after the workout is complete, aiding in weight loss and fat burning. Additionally, finisher sets help to improve muscular endurance by pushing muscles to perform under fatigue. This challenge strengthens the muscles and improves their ability to sustain activity over extended periods, ultimately enhancing overall stamina and endurance. Furthermore, finisher sets are highly time-efficient, providing an intense workout experience in a short amount of time. This makes them ideal for individuals with busy schedules who may struggle to find extended periods for exercise. Whether used to cap off a workout session or as a standalone routine, finisher sets offer a quick and effective way to maximize your efforts and achieve your fitness goals.

Incorporate finisher sets into your workout routine to challenge yourself, break through plateaus, and maximize the effectiveness of your training sessions. Adjust the exercises and intensity level based on your fitness level and goals, and always prioritize proper form and technique to prevent injury.

Do not underestimate the power of recovery. While it is not as active as pumping iron with occlusion bands on, planned recovery is a strategy for growth in and of itself. Adequate rest, including both sleep and non-exercise days, allows for muscle repair and growth. Additionally, stretching and mobility work can improve muscle function and overall BOT effectiveness (Laurent et al., 2020).

Tracking progress is more than just a motivational tool; it is a strategy for continued growth. Documenting workouts, including weights, exercise selection, band tightness, repetitions, and perceived effort, can provide valuable insights into what works for your body and what does not. Tweak your training based on this feedback to keep moving forward.

Combine BOT with other training modalities to prevent adaptation. The body is incredibly adept at adjusting to stress, so introducing new stimuli is necessary for growth. This could mean incorporating high-intensity interval training, plyometrics, or even endurance work on alternate days to your BOT routine.

Fueling your body correctly aligns perfectly with BOT for muscle growth. Nutrition plays a critical role and can amplify the effects of BOT. As you learned in the chapters above, a diet rich in protein, healthy fats, and adequate carbohydrates will provide the energy for workouts and the building blocks for muscle repair and growth. However, to help break through a plateau may entail boosting carbohydrate and calorie intake to provide muscles with added energy and kickstart metabolism. Hydration and the timing of nutrient intake can also play significant roles in your progress (Schoenfeld & Aragon, 2018).

Do not overlook the importance of mental strategies. Setting clear goals, maintaining a positive mindset, and visualizing success can enhance your physical training by keeping you motivated and focused. Mental toughness enables you to push through the discomfort associated with BOT and can lead to further growth.

Education is a never-ending process in the journey for muscle mastery. Keep learning about the latest research in exercise science, particularly concerning BOT. New studies are continually shedding light on the most effective ways to utilize this training method for maximum gains.

Understanding your body's signals is essential. If you are overtraining, experiencing excessive fatigue, or hitting a plateau despite all your efforts, it is time to reassess. Perhaps you need to adjust your overall intensity of your workouts and add in an extra rest day or "active rest" day, as mentioned in previous chapters.

It is about finding the perfect balance that challenges your muscles without leading to overtraining or injury.

Networking with other BOT practitioners and users can also present new strategies and insights. Sharing experiences and discussing successes and challenges can help refine your approach to BOT and stimulate continuous growth.

Lastly, always prioritize safety. While pursuing growth is important, it must never come at the cost of your health. Ensure that the application of BOT and all related training protocols adhere strictly to the recommended safety guidelines to prevent any adverse outcomes (Clark et al., 2011).

To summarize, strategies for continued growth in BOT involve a multifaceted approach that includes workout variability, periodization, intensity techniques, recovery, progress tracking, multimodal training, proper nutrition, mental strategies, continued education, body awareness, community engagement, and unwavering adherence to safety practices.

By implementing these strategies, you build not only muscle but also the resilience and adaptability necessary to maintain a trajectory of lifelong fitness and health success.

When to Increase Intensity in BOT

As you get deeper into the world of blood occlusion training (BOT), you may notice that your progress sometimes hits a plateau. This is a natural part of any fitness journey, but it is also a sign that your body is adapting to the current level of stress you are placing on it. To continue advancing your muscle mastery, it is crucial to recognize when it is time to increase the intensity of your BOT routines. In this section, we will explore the signs to look for and the best practices for safely ramping up your BOT sessions.

Understanding when to step up your game within BOT is more nuanced than simply adding more weight or time to your workouts. The unique nature of BOT—having to do with occlusion and blood flow modulation—requires a careful approach to intensifying your regimen. A key indicator that you are ready to move forward is when your current workout no longer leaves you with that characteristic "pump" or when muscle fatigue does not set in by the end of your session (Suga et al., 2012).

Another telltale sign is if you are able to comfortably complete all the repetitions and sets with a given occlusion pressure and weight without reaching near muscular failure. This comfort points towards your muscles having adapted to the demand, and hence, an increased intensity could be beneficial (Loenneke et al., 2011). Muscle soreness, although not always a reliable indicator, when it decreases consistently after consecutive workouts, may also suggest it is time for a change.

If you are tracking your performance metrics—and you should be—consistent improvements over time with no perceivable increase in effort can be a clue that your body has become more efficient under the current conditions. Monitoring factors such as repetition maximums, time under tension, and overall workout volume will guide your decision on when to turn up the intensity dial (Loenneke et al., 2012).

Furthermore, psychological readiness should not be ignored. When workouts start to feel monotonous and no longer challenge you mentally, the motivational benefits of increasing intensity can be just as important as the physiological ones. This mental plateau suggests you are ready for the next hurdle and can handle a boost in difficulty.

Once you have determined it is time to increase intensity, the question becomes how to do it safely. In BOT, this means manipulating variables like the duration of occlusion, volume of exercise (sets and repetitions), type of exercise, how much weight and recovery time between sets. However, never increase the tightness of the band; always maintain a consistent level of 7 out of 10 tightness. A conservative approach is to increase only one variable at a time while keeping others constant, to gauge how your body responds (Loenneke & Pujol, 2009).

The duration of occlusion is also an area where intensity can be adjusted. Extending the amount of time your limbs are occluded during rest periods can increase the metabolic stress and potential for muscle growth. However, it is critical not to extend occlusion to the point of discomfort or numbness, maintaining a balanced approach to health and safety. Therefore, do not leave the tourniquet on the upper limb for more than 15 mins and lower body no more than 20 mins at a time. (Takarada et al., 2000).

Adjusting the volume of exercise is one method for increasing intensity. Adding more sets or repetitions can lead to greater muscle fiber recruitment and hypertrophy, without needing to increase occlusion pressure (Pearson & Hussain, 2015). However, it is essential to pay attention to your body's recovery needs and avoid overtraining.

Changing the type of exercise is always a good move too. Instead of focusing on single muscle groups, such as the biceps, in bicep curls or quadriceps, in leg extensions, the intensity could be increased with a multi-muscle exercise. Recruiting multiple muscle groups at one time with a single exercise, such as squats by activating the whole leg would signal a greater muscle building response.

Increasing the weight, you are lifting is a traditional method of upping intensity, but within BOT, this should be done cautiously. Due to the occlusion effect, heavyweights are not necessary for achieving muscle growth. Therefore, slight increases in weight, along with careful monitoring of muscle response, is the way to proceed.

Finally, decreasing the recovery time between sets can enhance the intensity of your BOT workout. Shorter rest periods force the muscle to adapt to less recovery time, increasing the metabolic demand and potentially fostering greater endurance and hypertrophy (Laurentino et al., 2012).

While the discussion on increasing intensity is important, equally crucial is knowing what not to do. Avoid substantial increases in any of these variables all at once. This can lead to injury or counterproductive levels of fatigue. Moreover, do not disregard personal comfort and signs of excessive strain, as BOT should not elicit sharp pain or a loss of limb sensation.

To effectively and safely increase intensity in your blood occlusion training, it is advisable to keep a detailed training log, regularly assess your progression, and stay attuned to your body's responses. Engaging with a professional, such as a physical therapist or certified trainer knowledgeable in BOT, can provide personalized advice and supervision during this advancement phase.

Remember, while aiming to increase intensity to overcome plateaus, the overarching goal is to continue to make sustainable, safe gains. Every individual's journey with BOT will be distinct, and so should their intensity adjustments. With a strategic, informed approach, you will keep moving forward, continuing to trick your body into believing it is undergoing more intense workouts than it actually is, promoting real,

lasting muscle growth without overstressing the

system.

Recovery Principles to Maximize Muscle Gains

Nutrition and recovery are critical components in any training program, and this holds especially true when discussing accelerated muscle building and breaking through plateaus. The process of muscle hypertrophy is not solely reliant on what happens during training but is equally dependent on what occurs after the weights are put down. This section educates the fundamental principles of recovery, emphasizing its significance in the realm of blood occlusion training (BOT).

Blood occlusion training, by its nature, presents a unique challenge to muscle recovery. This innovative technique restricts blood flow to working muscles, creating an environment that fosters significant muscular gains without the need for heavy weights.

When practicing BOT, understanding and implementing robust recovery strategies becomes paramount.

As discussed in the previous chapters, muscle recovery begins with proper nutrition, sleep, and hydration. However, it needs to be mentioned again that consuming adequate amounts of protein is of utmost importance as it supplies the amino acids needed for repair and growth of muscle tissue (Phillips & Van Loon, 2011). Coupled with BOT, a diet rich in quality protein can significantly boost muscle synthesis rates during the critical post-workout window.

Furthermore, carbohydrates also play a vital role in recovery as they replenish muscle glycogen stores that have been depleted during exercise. Incorporating a balanced amount of carbohydrates post-workout can improve recovery and aid in the process of muscle building, particularly when paired with protein (Ivy, 2004).

Another powerful tool is active recovery methods, such as light aerobic exercise or mobility work. This can enhance circulation and promote muscle repair without imposing additional stress on the muscle fibers. These techniques are particularly synergistic with BOT as they assist the removal of metabolic byproducts associated with the localized hypoxic condition (Fujita et al., 2007).

The application of compression garments, such as compression sleeves or compression pants may offer additional benefits in muscle recovery. These garments can help reduce exercise-induced swelling and perceived muscle soreness, potentially leading to a faster recovery process which can be highly advantageous following BOT sessions (Kraemer et al., 2001).

Recovery is not just a physical process; it is also psychological. Mental stress can play a detrimental role in an individual's ability to recover. Techniques geared towards stress reduction, like meditation or deep-breathing exercises, can improve overall recovery by promoting a more anabolic environment for muscle growth.

The timing of recovery interventions also merits attention. Post-exercise nutrition, for instance, is most impactful when consumed soon after a workout. This is often termed the "anabolic window," a period where the body is primed to utilize nutrients for repair and growth at an accelerated rate (Schoenfeld et al., 2013).

Finally, recovery is highly individualized; what works for one person might not be as effective for another. Personalizing recovery strategies, especially in the context of BOT, is vital. Listen to your body and adapt recovery practices based on personal response and muscle adaptation.

To sum up, recovery is not merely a passive phase but an active component of muscle building, particularly in programs incorporating blood occlusion training. Proper nutrition, adequate hydration, sufficient rest, active recovery techniques, psychological stress management, and the astute timing of interventions work harmoniously to maximize muscle gains. Embracing these recovery principles will ensure that each training session is built upon a strong foundation, leading to more efficient and accelerated muscle growth.

By meticulously applying these recovery and plateau principles, anyone from fitness enthusiasts, athletes, military personnel, to the elderly and injured can capitalize on the benefits of BOT. Also, breaking through plateaus and navigating towards unprecedented gains in muscle strength and size.

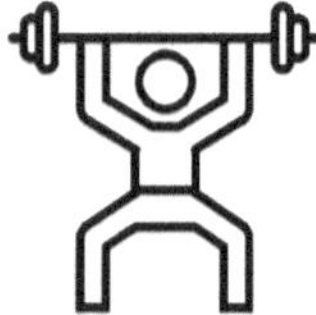

Conclusion

mbracing the journey to Muscle Mastery is not merely about achieving a momentary goal but rather about taking a transformative journey—one that challenges both body and mind. We have journeyed together through the science and methodologies of Blood Occlusion Training (BOT), learning how this approach can lead to incredible strength and muscle gains without demanding heavy weights or excessive time commitments. Now, it is about carrying forward the lessons learned and embracing the path to continual improvement.

Our exploration of BOT opened with an understanding of its mechanisms, allowing us to see how muscle growth can be facilitated through strategic occlusion. With this knowledge, we dove into procedures and case studies that illuminated the method's efficacy across a range of individuals—from athletes and military personnel to those recovering from injuries.

Special populations, including the elderly and amputees, were not left out of the equation. In tailoring BOT to their unique needs, we have seen how inclusivity in fitness not only benefits physical health but also boosts longevity and quality of life by increasing muscle strength. All this was accomplished while keeping safety at the cornerstone of our discovery, ensuring that the practices adopted serve the end-user without incurring undue risk.

Overcoming plateaus is a crucial aspect of any training regimen, and in Chapter 9, strategies for ongoing growth kept us focused on the horizon. Increasing intensity with BOT is a nuanced decision, but you now possess the insights necessary to decide

when and how to safely ramp up your training efforts.

We also delved into the vital roles of nutrition,

reading food labels and how to meal prep.

Understanding the significance of reading food labels

and incorporating meal prepping into one's routine is

pivotal for achieving successful muscle building goals.

Together, these practices empower individuals to take

control of their diet, maximize muscle-building

potential, and ultimately achieve their fitness objectives

more efficiently. Building muscle is not only about

lifting weights; it also requires careful attention to

nutrition, and by prioritizing reading food labels and

meal prepping, individuals can lay a solid foundation

for success in their muscle-building journey. As you

have come to understand, building muscle is a holistic

endeavor; one must fuel the body appropriately to maximize gains from BOT.

We have also emphasized the critical importance of prioritizing muscle recovery and injury prevention, which is paramount for both athletes and fitness enthusiasts. Recovery is not just a time of rest—it is a period of potentiation for your muscles to regrow stronger and more resilient. By incorporating proper rest, nutrition, and recovery techniques into training regimens, individuals can optimize their performance, reduce the risk of injuries, and promote long-term health and well-being. Moreover, paying attention to warning signs of fatigue or discomfort and adjusting training intensity accordingly can help prevent more serious injuries down the line. Ultimately, by fostering a holistic approach to training that encompasses both physical and mental well-being, individuals can enjoy sustainable progress and achieve their fitness goals safely and effectively.

As we close this chapter, it is important to reflect on the journey that muscle mastery truly is. It is filled with highs and lows, triumphs and challenges. The key is to stay the course, applying the principles of BOT consistently and with patience.

Remember, mastery is not just about physical prowess; it is about the deep understanding and connection to the process. It is about the attention to detail that you incorporated when you were learning about BOT—recognizing how slight adjustments can make substantial differences in your results.

Moreover, the journey to muscle mastery is personal and ever evolving. As you grow and adapt, so too will your training. BOT offers a framework, but it is your dedication, effort, and willingness to listen to your body that will ultimately drive your success.

Consider how this journey has expanded beyond the gym walls. The disciplines learned have likely spilled over into other areas of your life, enhancing discipline, mental fortitude, and the relentless pursuit of personal excellence.

Engaging with BOT is about smart training, not just hard training. It is crucial to remember that the quality of your workouts is paramount—using the principles of occlusion to strategically trigger muscle growth and strength gains in ways that past training methods may not have achieved.

For the skeptics turned believers, your transformed perspective through scientific understanding hopefully serves as inspiration for others who may still be hesitant to embrace such a novel approach to training. The empirical evidence has served as a foundation, but your testimonies and achievements will carry the message further. As you continue on your path, share what you have learned with others. The power of community in the fitness realm cannot be overstated. By being a part of the BOT conversation, you are paving the way for newcomers and providing insights that can only be gained through experience. Share your enthusiasm about BOT with others to help them in their journey. Please write a review on this book to help get the message out on how Blood Occlusion Training really works!

Looking ahead, your journey does not end here. It is a continuous cycle of learning, applying, adjusting, and advancing. Keep abreast of new research and developments in BOT and related fields to refine your approach and find novel ways to enhance your training. In the spirit of this ongoing journey, your final takeaway from this book is to embrace every step of your muscle mastery quest with curiosity, commitment, and the confidence that comes from knowing you are on a scientifically proven path to achieving your fitness aspirations. To your strength, resilience, and relentless progress—may you continue to thrive in the pursuit of muscle mastery through a healthy lifestyle and Blood Occlusion Training.

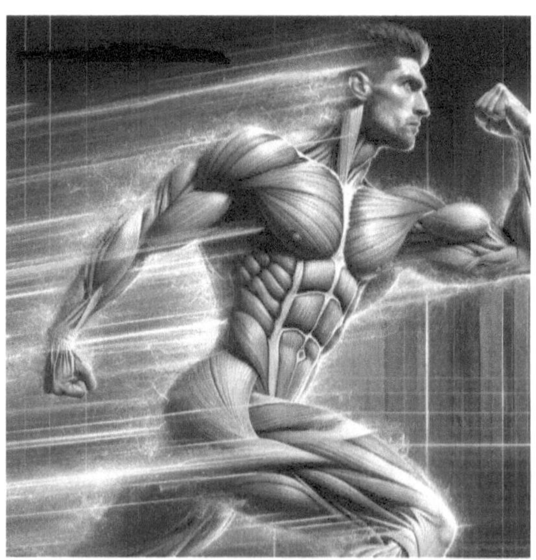

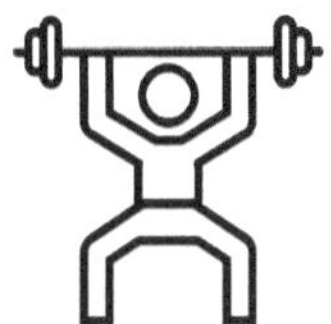

Blood Occlusion Protocol Cheat Sheet

When diving into blood occlusion training (BOT), it is critical to get the basics right to ensure both safety and effectiveness. Here is a cheat sheet to help you ace the protocol.

Protocol:

- **Placement and Tightness:** Secure the tourniquet as high as possible on the limb being trained. For arms, this means at the uppermost bicep area, and for legs, it is right below the buttocks. Remember, it should not be a pain-fest; you are going for a snug fit, with a perceived tightness of about 7 out of 10. If it is causing pain before starting or hindering your ability to perform reps, loosen it up a tad.

- **Exercise Protocol:** Athletes, military personnel, fitness enthusiasts, and post-op musculoskeletal surgery patients, as well as amputees, will go for 30 reps at 20-30% of their 1RM, then cruise through 3 sets of 15 reps, with a brief 30 second rest between sets, engaging in this routine 2-3 times a week. This is not about lifting the heaviest weights but creating the significant tension that promotes muscle growth (Loenneke et al., 2012).

- **Walking Protocol:** A 20-minute treadmill walk at a gentle 2.5 mph can be paired with BFR to make those muscles work smarter. Keeping the restriction pressure of the blood pressure cuff dialed in at 160 to 200 mmHg for a 20-minute stretch helps maintain the balance between safety and efficacy and ensures that elderly and amputees see results without going overboard (Patterson & Brandner, 2018).

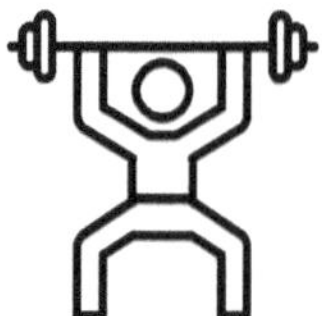

Week 1-2: Beginner Exercises

Upper Body: Bicep Curl, Tricep Extension

Lower Body: Leg Extension, Hamstring Curl

* Choose one exercise and complete the exercise by itself following the BOT protocol: 30 reps at 20-30% of 1RM, then 3 sets of 15 reps, with a brief 30 second rest between sets. If feeling motivated, add ONE more exercise for the same body category and then immediately take the tourniquet off as soon as the exercises are finished. Warning: Do not keep the occlusion band on for more than 5-10 mins.

** Complete the upper body one day and the next day move onto the lower body with one rest day in between. Rotate this for 2 weeks or until a plateau has been reached which has been discussed earlier in this book and then move onto the advanced section.

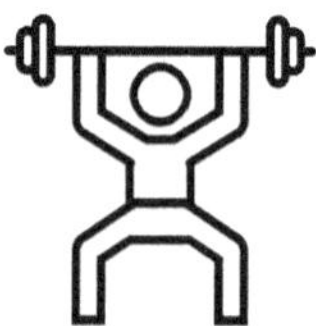

Instructions on How to Complete Each Beginner Exercise:

Bicep Curl:

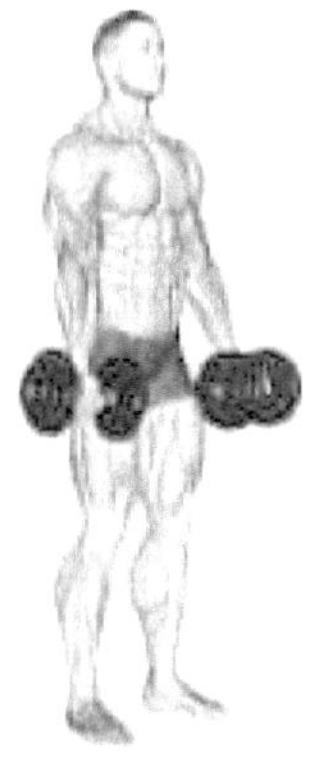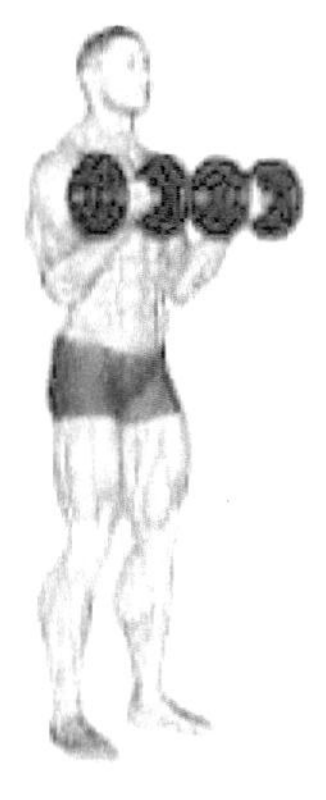

Stand with your feet shoulder-width apart, hold either a dumbbell in each hand, TheraBand or barbell with palms facing up. With a straight posture and engaged core, initiate the exercise by bending your elbows while keeping them close to your body. As you do this, lift the weights towards your shoulders in a controlled manner. Focus on squeezing your biceps to maximize the contraction. Then, in a controlled manner, lower the weights back to the starting position. It is essential to maintain proper form throughout the exercise, avoiding any swinging or momentum. Do not forget to breathe: Exhale while lifting, inhale while lowering.

Tricep Extension:

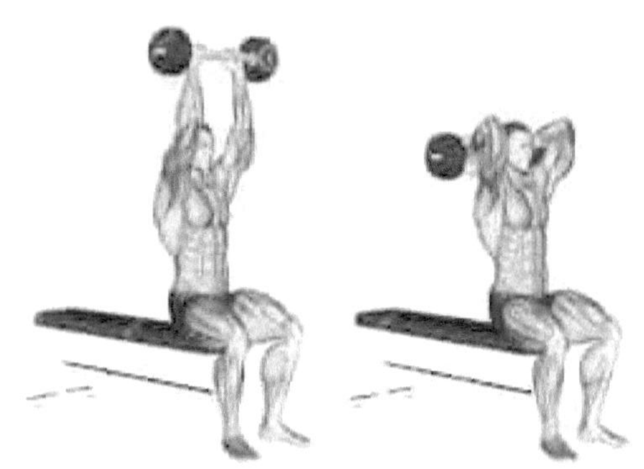

Stand or sit with proper posture. Hold a dumbbell with both hands above your head. Lower the dumbbell behind your head by bending your elbows; your upper arms should stay close to your ears. Then, extend your arms upward, straightening your elbows fully. Concentrate on contracting your triceps as you push the weight upward. Once elbows are fully extended, slowly return to the starting position. Repeat this movement for the desired number of repetitions.

Throughout the exercise, maintain core engagement to stabilize your body and ensure controlled execution.

Leg Extension:

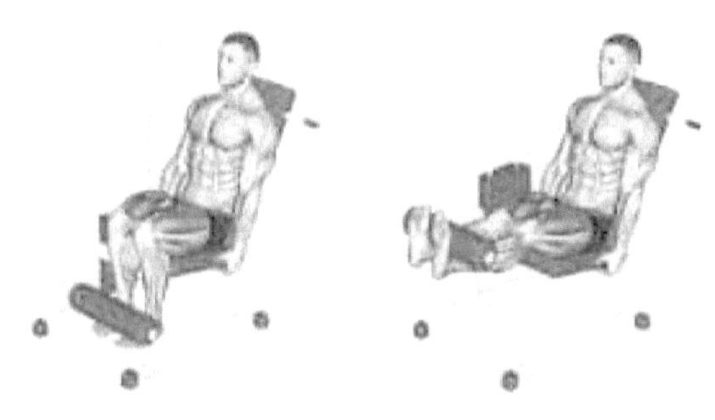

Sit on a leg extension machine with your back against the backrest and your feet securely positioned under the padded roller. Grasp the handles on the sides of the machine for stability. Extend your legs fully, lifting the padded roller until your legs are straight. Focus on contracting your quadriceps at the top of the movement, and then slowly lower the weight back to the starting position by bending your knees. Control the weight, avoiding jerking motions and locking of the knees. Repeat for the desired number of repetitions. This could also be performed at home using light ankle weights as well.

Hamstring Curl:

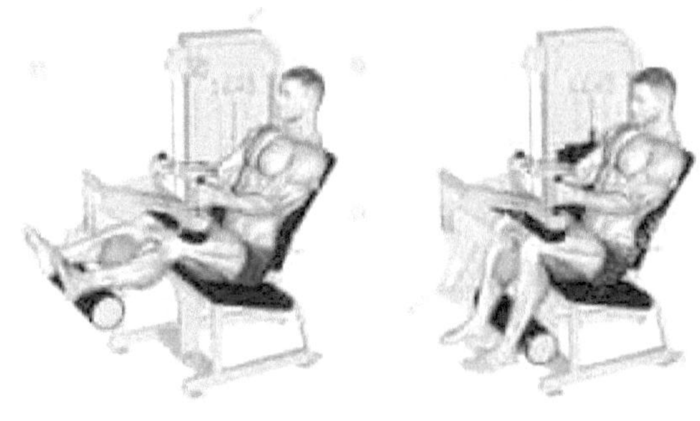

Lay face down or seated on a leg curl machine (depends which machine is available) with your legs fully extended and the padded roller resting against your ankles. Grasp the handles for support. Begin by bending your knees as far as comfortably possible, focusing on contracting your hamstrings. Slowly return the weight to the starting position, extending your legs fully. Maintain a controlled pace. Perform the hamstring curl for the desired number of repetitions.

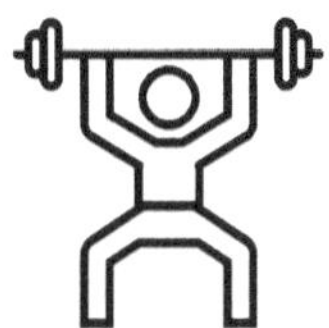

Week 3-4: <u>Advanced Exercises</u>

Upper Body: Shoulder Press, Chest Press, Lateral Shoulder Raise, Seated Rows

Lower Body: Squat, Split Lunge, Lateral Squat Walk, Single-Leg Deadlift, Calf Raise

* To start off choose one exercise and complete the exercise by itself following the BOT protocol: 30 reps at 20-30% of 1RM, then 3 sets of 15 reps, with a brief 30 second rest between sets. If feeling motivated, add ONE more exercise for the SAME body category and then immediately take the tourniquet off as soon as the exercises are finished. Warning: Do not keep the occlusion band on for more than 10-20 mins.

** With the tourniquet on complete a max of 2 upper body exercises one day and the next day complete a max of 2 lower body exercises with one rest day in between. Rotate this for 2 weeks or until a plateau has been reached. These advanced exercises are just a starting tool and an example of what can be done with BOT. The ADVANCED EXERCISES can be performed with the traditional BOT protocol or as follows with or without the tourniquet on preformed as a **drop set** (an exercise performed until muscle failure, then quickly reduce the weight and continue lifting), a **super set** (perform two different opposing exercises back-to-back with little or no rest in between) or a **finisher set** (perform a regular workout without BOT, then finish the workout with the traditional BOT protocol for the same muscle group just worked).

Here is a detailed example of a **drop set** using the dumbbell bicep curl exercise: Begin by selecting a pair of dumbbells, typically 70-80% of your one-repetition maximum (1RM) for bicep curls. Perform repetitions until reaching momentary muscular failure. Without resting, immediately switch to lighter dumbbells, around 50-60% of initial weight. Continue bicep curls with lighter dumbbells until reaching failure again. Repeat process, reducing weight and performing additional repetitions until unable to lift dumbbells with proper form. Allow biceps to fully recover before targeting the same muscle group again.

A thorough explanation of a **superset** regimen using the bench press and seated row is: Perform the bench press exercise for the prescribed number of repetitions. Immediately transition to the bent-over rows exercise without resting. Perform the bent-over rows for the prescribed number of repetitions. Rest for 60-90 seconds after completing both exercises in the superset. Repeat the superset for the desired number of sets, typically 3-4 sets.

The procedure for a **finisher set** is: Perform each exercise in the circuit consecutively, completing as many repetitions as possible within the specified time frame (30 seconds per exercise). Rest for 30 seconds between exercises or transition directly from one exercise to the next for maximum intensity. Complete the entire circuit for 2-3 rounds, depending on your fitness level and energy levels. Focus on maintaining proper form and intensity throughout the finisher set, pushing yourself to work at maximum effort to fully fatigue the muscles and elevate the heart rate.

Examples of a **Finisher set** using Bodyweight Exercises:

Jump Squats after weighted squats:

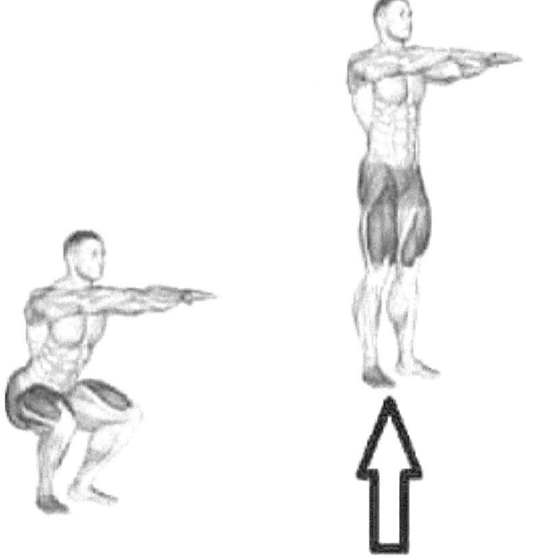

Start in a standing position with your feet shoulder-width apart. Lower your body into a squat position by bending your knees and pushing your hips back. Explosively jump upward, extending your legs fully. Land softly and immediately lower back into a squat position to begin the next repetition. Perform as many jump squats as possible within 30 seconds, focusing on explosiveness and maintaining proper form.

Push-Ups after bench press:

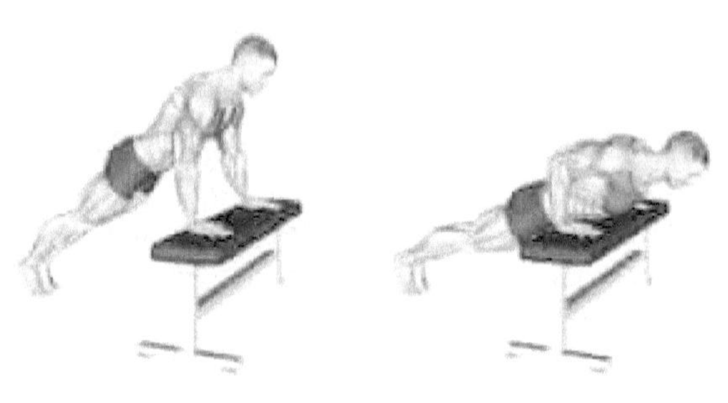

Begin in a high plank position with your hands placed slightly wider than shoulder-width apart, arms fully extended, and body forming a straight line from head to heels. Lower your body towards the floor or bench by bending your elbows, keeping them close to your sides. Lower until your chest nearly touches the ground or bench, then push through your palms to return to the starting position. Perform as many push-ups as possible within 30 seconds, focusing on maintaining a strong core and full range of motion. Utilizing a bench, as illustrated in the picture, can be beneficial in making the exercise more manageable and allow for increased repetitions.

Pull-ups after bicep curls:

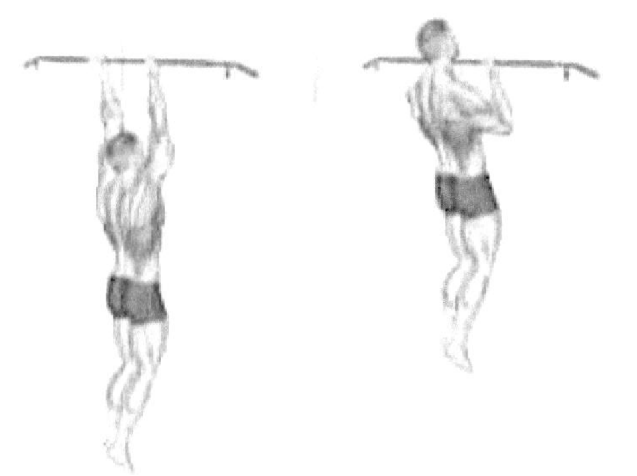

Grab an overhead bar with an underhand grip, hands slightly wider than shoulder-width apart. Hang from the bar with arms fully extended and feet off the ground. Engage your back and bicep muscles and pull your body upward until your chin clears the bar. Lower yourself back down with control until your arms are fully extended. Repeat for the desired number of repetitions, focusing on maintaining proper form throughout the movement. Utilizing a band for assistance or relying on a pull-up machine can be beneficial if performing a pull-up independently is difficult.

Now is your turn to get creative! Mix up the exercises and the sequence on how you perform them to help prevent plateaus and injury. Remember, this cheat sheet is a guide to get you started on BOT, but do not shy away from digging into the concepts and principles discussed in previous chapters. It is about training smarter, not necessarily harder, and this method is all about efficiency while keeping an eye on safety.

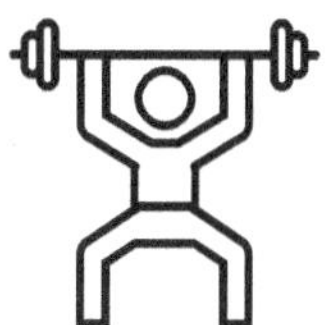

Instructions on How to Complete Each Advanced Exercise:

Shoulder Press:

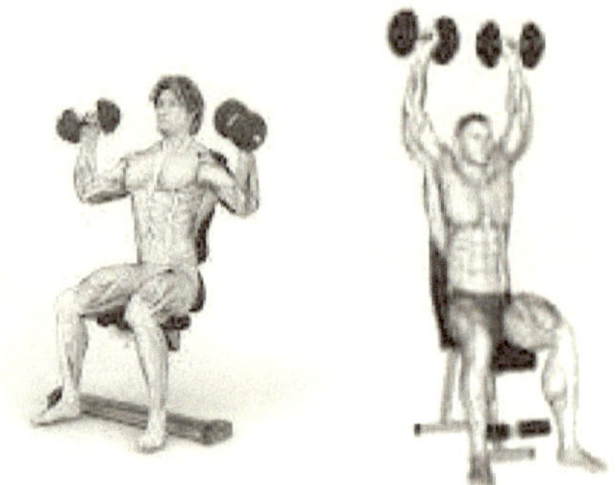

Sit or stand with your back straight and core engaged. Hold a dumbbell in each hand at shoulder height, with your palms facing forward and elbows bent. Push the weights upward by extending your arms fully overhead until the weights almost touch at the top. Focus on engaging your shoulder muscles during this upward motion. Lower the weights back down to shoulder level in a controlled manner by bending your elbows. Repeat this movement for the desired number of repetitions, ensuring a steady and controlled pace throughout.

Chest Press:

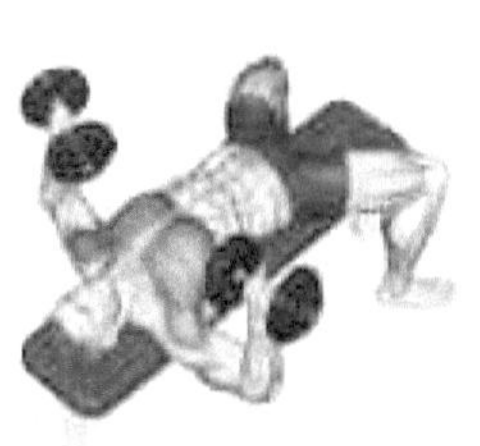 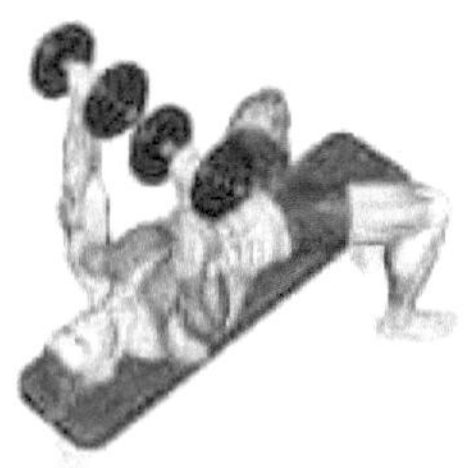

Lie flat on a bench with your back pressed firmly against it. Hold a dumbbell in each hand above your chest, with your palms facing away from you and your elbows bent at a 90-degree angle. Push the dumbbells upward, extending your arms fully until the weights nearly touch at the top. Contract your chest muscles. Lower the dumbbells back down to chest level in a controlled manner by bending your elbows. Perform this motion for the desired number of repetitions, maintaining a controlled pace and ensuring that your back remains on the bench throughout.

Lateral Shoulder Raise:

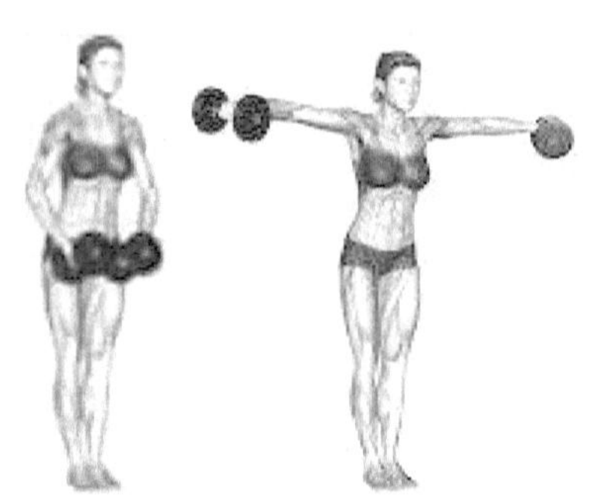

Stand with your feet shoulder-width apart, holding a dumbbell in each hand by your sides with your palms facing your body. Keep a slight bend in your elbows. Maintaining this position, lift both dumbbells out to your sides until they reach shoulder level, forming a "T" shape with your arms. Focus on engaging your shoulder muscles during this motion. Lower the dumbbells back down to your sides in a controlled manner. Repeat this movement for the desired number of repetitions, ensuring a controlled pace and avoiding swinging or using momentum.

Seated Row:

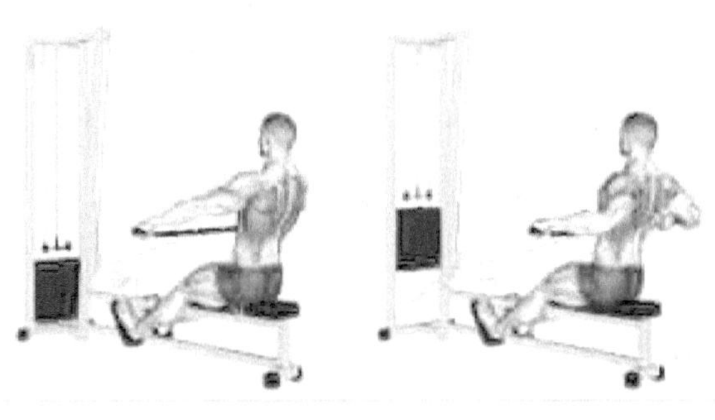 Sit on a rowing machine or a bench with your feet flat on the floor and your knees slightly bent. Grasp the handle or the attachment in front of you with both hands, keeping your palms facing each other. Keep your back straight, shoulders relaxed, and core engaged. Start by pulling the handle or attachment toward your lower chest, squeezing your shoulder blades together as you do so. Your elbows should be close to your body. Slowly return the handle to the starting position, fully extending your arms. Repeat this motion for the desired number of repetitions,

maintaining a controlled pace and focusing on using your back muscles for the pull.

Squat:

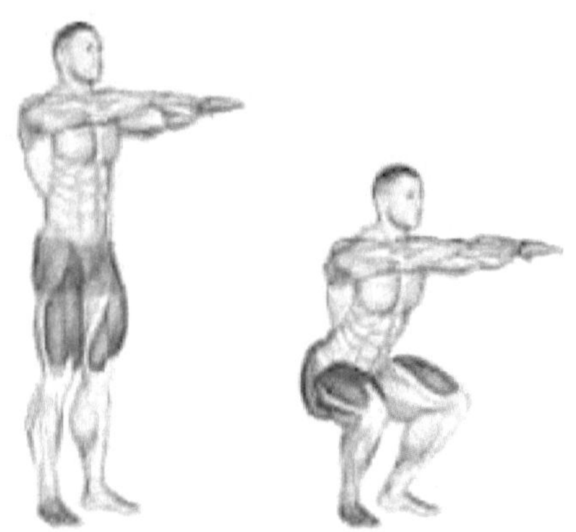

Stand with your feet shoulder-width apart, chest up, and core engaged. Lower your body by bending your knees and hips, as if you are sitting back into a chair. Keep your back straight and chest up as you lower yourself. Go down until your thighs are parallel to the ground or as far as your flexibility allows. Push through your heels to return to the standing position. Keep your knees aligned with your feet throughout the movement. Squats effectively target your leg muscles, particularly your quads, hamstrings, and glutes, while also engaging your core for stability.

Split Lunge:

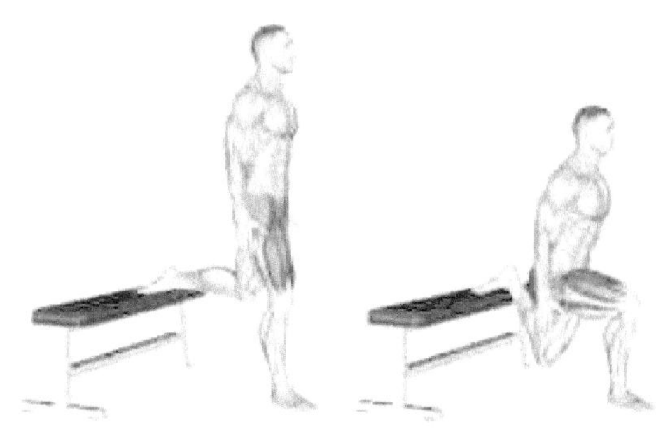

Stand with your feet together. Step one foot forward and one foot backward, creating a split stance. To make it more difficult, your back foot can be resting on a bench (shown) or step. Bend your knees to lower your body, with the front knee forming a 90-degree angle. Your front knee should be aligned with your ankle, and your back knee should hover just above the ground. Keep your upper body upright with good posture. Push through your front heel to return to the starting position. Alternate between legs for repetitions. Split lunges are an effective lower body exercise that targets your quadriceps, hamstrings, and glutes while also engaging your core for balance.

Lateral Squat Walk:

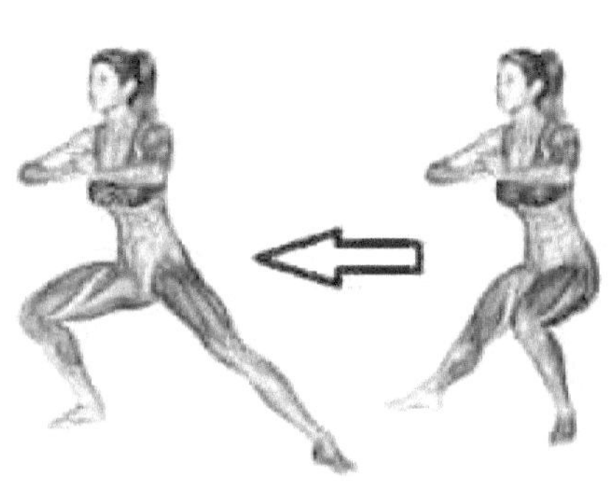

Stand with your feet hip-width apart, chest up, and core engaged (Perform with or without TheraBand around knees (easier) or ankles (harder). Lower your body into a squat position, hold the squat form as you take a step to the side with your right foot. Push off with your left foot and take a step to the side with your right foot, staying low in the squat. Continue this lateral squat walk pattern until all repetitions are completed to the right side then repeat to the left side. Maintain good posture throughout. Lateral squat walks are excellent for working your leg muscles, particularly the inner and outer thighs, while also improving hip mobility and stability.

Single-Leg Deadlift:

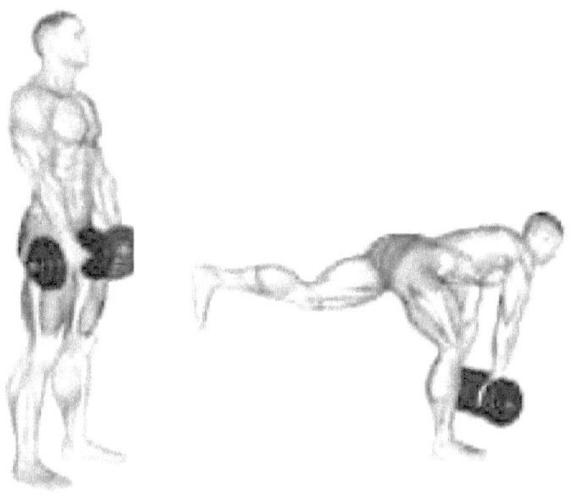

Stand on one leg with a slight bend in the knee. Hold a dumbbell or kettlebell in one hand with your arm extended down in front of you. While keeping your back straight and shoulders back, hinge at your hips and lower your upper body forward as you lift your non-standing leg straight behind you. Continue lowering until your upper body and non-standing leg are parallel to the ground, creating a straight line from head to heel. Engage your glutes and hamstrings as you return to the starting position. Maintain balance and control throughout the movement. Single-leg deadlifts target the hamstrings, glutes, and lower back while also enhancing balance and stability.

Calf Raise:

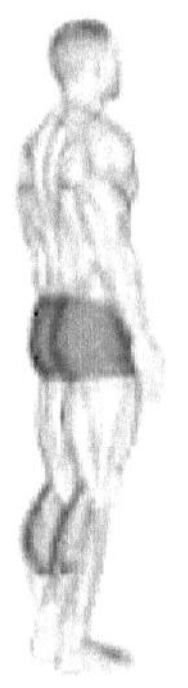 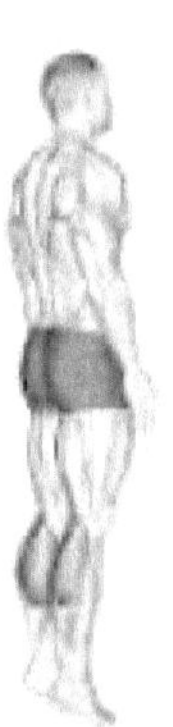

Stand upright with your feet hip-width apart. You can do this exercise with bodyweight,

holding onto a stable surface or using a calf raise

machine or a step. If using a step, place the balls of your feet on the edge of the step with your heels hanging off. Slowly raise your heels as high as you can by pushing through the balls of your feet, flexing your calf muscles at the top. Hold this position briefly, then lower your heels below the level of the step to get a full stretch in your calf muscles. Perform the desired number of repetitions, aiming for a full range of motion and controlled movement. Calf raises are an effective exercise for strengthening the calf muscles and improving lower leg stability.

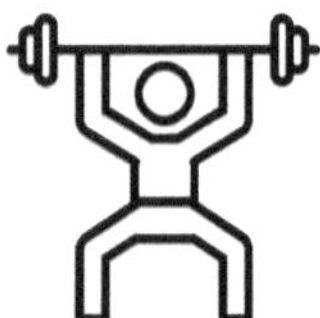

About the Author

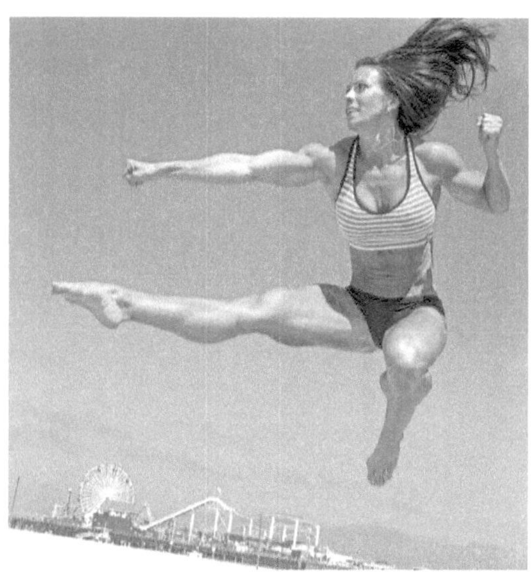

The author brings a unique blend of academic expertise and personal experience to the world of fitness. With a background in physical therapy, she delved deep into the science of blood occlusion during her studies, even dedicating her thesis to this groundbreaking method. But it does not stop there – she is not just a scholar; she is a bodybuilder who has walked the walk. The author personally harnessed the power of blood occlusion to gain that coveted edge in their own fitness journey, even using it as a secret weapon in preparation for a bodybuilding competition. As you can see in the image above, the results speak for themselves. Thanks to her profound knowledge and practical application of blood occlusion, she has been able to fast-track her way to achieving remarkable fitness goals.

Ending Remarks

As an author and fitness professional, one of the greatest joys is knowing that my book and guidance has resonated with readers like you. If you enjoyed reading my book and found value in its pages, I kindly ask for your assistance in spreading the word. If you have a moment to spare, please consider leaving a review by following this link or scanning the QR code provided below. Your words have the power to shape the future of this book and influence the lives of others who may come across it.

Book Link:

https://www.amazon.com/review/create-review/?ie=UTF8&channel=glance-detail&asin=B0CW1HBPR3

QR Code:

290

References

1. Abe, T., Kearns, C. F., & Sato, Y. (2006). Muscle size and strength are increased following walk training with restricted venous blood flow from the leg muscle, Kaatsu-walk training. Journal of Applied Physiology, 100(5), 1460-1466.

2. Abe, T., Sakamaki, M., Fujita, S., Ozaki, H., Sugaya, M., & Sato, Y. (2010). Effects of Low-Intensity Walk Training With Restricted Leg Blood Flow on Muscle Strength and Aerobic Capacity in Older Adults. Journal of Geriatric Physical Therapy, 33(1), 34–40.

3. Alhazmi, A., Kuriakose, B., & Muzammil, K. (2023). Prevalence, attitudes, and practices of dietary supplements among middle-aged and older adults in Asir region, Saudi Arabia: A cross-sectional study. PLoS One, 18(10), e0292900.

4. Brooks, K. (2018). The Effect of Ballistic Stretching on Flexibility and Performance. Journal of Applied Physiology, 124(2), 154-159.

5. Charge, S. B., & Rudnicki, M. A. (2004). Cellular and molecular regulation of muscle regeneration. Physiological Reviews, 84(1), 209-238.

6. Chen, J., Zhu, Q., Yu, L., Li, Y., Jia, S., Zhang, J., & Zhang, J. (2022). Stroke Risk Factors of Stroke Patients in China: A Nationwide Community-Based Cross-Sectional Study. International Journal of Environmental Research and Public Health, 19(8), 4807.

7. Cheuvront, S. N., & Kenefick, R. W. (2014). Dehydration: Physiology, Assessment, and Performance Effects. Sports Medicine, 44(S1), 155–161. https://doi.org/10.1007/s40279-014-0149-

8. Clark, D. R., Lambert, M. I., & Hunter, A. M. (2011). Muscle activation in the loaded free barbell squat: A brief review. Journal of Strength and Conditioning Research, 25(4), 1169-1178.

9. Cook, C. J., Kilduff, L. P., & Beaven, C. M. (2014). Improving strength and power in trained athletes with 3 weeks of occlusion training. International Journal of Sports Physiology and Performance, 9(1), 166-172.

10. Dattilo, M., Antunes, H. K., Medeiros, A., Mônico Neto, M., Souza, H. S., Tufik, S., & de Mello, M. T. (2011). Sleep and muscle recovery: Endocrinological and molecular basis for a new and promising hypothesis. Medical Hypotheses, 77(2), 220-222.

11. Effects of exercise with and without different degrees of blood flow restriction on torque and muscle activation - Clinical Medicine - Popular Study. (n.d.). Retrieved January 17, 2015, from http://medicine.popularstudy.com/stories/1171 54/Effects_of_exercise_with_and_without_diff erent_degrees_of_blood_flow_restriction_on_t orque_and_muscle_activation.html

12. Fernandez, J. (2021). Myofascial Release as a Tool for Recovery: A Systematic Review. International Journal of Sports Medicine, 42(3), 196-203.

13. Fry, A. C. (2004). The role of resistance exercise intensity on muscle fibre adaptations. Sports Medicine, 34(10), 663-679.

14. Fujita, S., Abe, T., Drummond, M. J., Cadenas, J. G., Dreyer, H. C., Sato, Y., ... & Rasmussen, B. B.

(2007). Blood flow restriction during low-intensity resistance exercise increases S6K1 phosphorylation and muscle protein synthesis. Journal of Applied Physiology, 103(3), 903-910.

15. Houston, D. K., Nicklas, B. J., & Ding, J. (2008). Dietary protein intake is associated with lean mass change in older, community-dwelling adults: the Health, Aging, and Body Composition (Health ABC) Study. American Journal of Clinical Nutrition, 87(1), 150-155.

16. Ivy, J. L. (2004). Regulation of muscle glycogen repletion, muscle protein synthesis and repair following exercise. Journal of Sports Science & Medicine, 3(3), 131.

17. Improving Recovery with PNF Techniques. (2023, April 10). Fittr. https://www.fittr.com/articles/improving-recovery-with-pnf/

18. Johnson, D., & Anderson, F. (2020). The role of warm-up in muscular injury prevention. American Journal of Sports Medicine, 48(4), 1239-1252.

19. Johnson, G., & Johnson, P. (2021). Dynamic Stretching and Its Impact on Muscular Performance. European Journal of Sports Science, 21(1), 100-108.

20. Johnson, S., & Smith, M. (2012). The effects of static stretching on running performance. European Journal of Sport Science, 12(2), 100-105.

21. Jones, L. (2020). Portion control in meal prepping: Its significance in weight management. Journal of Nutritional Health, 15(3), 122-129.

22. Kacin, A., & Strazar, K. (2011). Frequent low-load ischemic resistance exercise to failure enhances muscle oxygen delivery and endurance capacity. Scandinavian Journal of Medicine & Science in Sports, 21(6), e231-e241.

23. Karabulut, M., Abe, T., Sato, Y., & Bemben, M. G. (2010). The effects of low-intensity resistance training with vascular restriction on leg muscle strength in older men. European Journal of Applied Physiology, 108(1), 147-155.

24. Kraemer, W. J., Bush, J. A., Wickham, R. B., Denegar, C. R., Gómez, A. L., Gotshalk, L. A., ... & Volek, J. S. (2001). Influence of compression therapy on symptoms following soft tissue injury from maximal eccentric exercise. The Journal of Orthopaedic and Sports Physical Therapy, 31(6), 282-290.

25. Kreider, R. B., Kalman, D. S., Antonio, J., Ziegenfuss, T. N., Wildman, R., Collins, R., ... & Lopez, H. L. (2017). International Society of Sports Nutrition position stand: safety and efficacy of creatine supplementation in exercise, sport, and medicine. Journal of the International Society of Sports Nutrition, 14(1), 18. https://doi.org/10.1186/s12970-017-0173-z

26. Kubota, A., Sakuraba, K., Sawaki, K., Sumide, T., & Tamura, Y. (2008). Prevention of disuse muscular weakness by restriction of blood flow. Medicine & Science in Sports & Exercise, 40(3), 529-534.

27. Laurent, C. M., Green, J. M., Bishop, P. A., Sjokvist, J., Schumacker, R. E., Richardson, M. T., & Curtner-Smith, M. (2020). Effect of rest duration on strength recovery in blood flow-

restricted resistance-trained muscle. Journal of Strength and Conditioning Research, 34(1), 1-7.

28. Laurentino, G., Ugrinowitsch, C., Aihara, A. Y., Fernandes, A. R., Parcell, A. C., Tricoli, V., & Roschel, H. (2008). Effects of Strength Training and Vascular Occlusion. International Journal of Sports Medicine, 29(8), 664–667; 33(07), 600-605; 33(8), 664–667.

29. Laurentino, G., Ugrinowitsch, C., Roschel, H., Aoki, M. S., Soares, A. G., Neves Jr, M., ... & Tricoli, V. (2012). Strength training with blood flow restriction diminishes myostatin gene expression. Medicine & Science in Sports & Exercise, 44(3), 406-412.

30. Lejkowski, Kin, & Pajaczkowski (2011). Utilization of Vascular Restriction Training in post-surgical knee rehabilitation: a case report and introduction to an under-reported training technique. Journal of the Canadian Chiropractic Association, 55(4), 280–287.

31. Lixandrão, M. E., Ugrinowitsch, C., Berton, R., Vechin, F. C., Conceição, M. S., Damas, F., Libardi, C. A., & Roschel, H. (2018). Magnitude

of muscle strength and mass adaptations between high-load resistance training versus low-load resistance training associated with blood-flow restriction: A systematic review and meta-analysis. Sports Medicine, 48(2), 361-378.

32. Loenneke, J. P., & Pujol, T. J. (2009). The Use of Occlusion Training to Produce Muscle Hypertrophy. Strength and Conditioning Journal, 31(3), 77–84.

33. Loenneke, J. P., Fahs, C. A., Rossow, L. M., Abe, T., & Bemben, M. G. (2012). The anabolic benefits of venous blood flow restriction training may be induced by muscle cell swelling. Medical Hypotheses, 78(1), 151-154.

34. Loenneke, J. P., Fahs, C. A., Rossow, L. M., Abe, T., Bemben, M. G. (2012). Effects of cuff width on arterial occlusion: implications for blood flow restricted exercise. European Journal of Applied Physiology, 112, 2903-2912.

35. Loenneke, J. P., Wilson, J. M., & Wilson, G. J. (2010). A mechanistic approach to blood flow occlusion. International Journal of Sports Medicine, 31(1), 1-4.

36. Loenneke, J. P., Wilson, J. M., Wilson, G. J., Pujol, T. J., & Bemben, M. G. (2012). Potential safety issues with blood flow restriction training. Scandinavian Journal of Medicine & Science in Sports, 22(4), 510-518.

37. Loenneke, J., Thiebaud, R., Abe, T., & Bemben, M. (2014). Blood flow restriction pressure recommendations: The hormesis hypothesis. Medical Hypotheses, 83, 623-626.

38. Loenneke, J.P., Fahs, C.A., Wilson, J.M., & Bemben, M.G. (2014). Blood flow restriction: The metabolite/volume threshold theory. Medical Hypotheses, 82(6), 748-752.

39. Loenneke, J.P., Wilson, J.M., Marín, P.J., Zourdos, M.C., & Bemben, M.G. (2012). Low-intensity blood flow restriction training: A meta-analysis. European Journal of Applied Physiology, 112(5), 1849-1859.

40. Laustsen, S. (2023, July 18). *The Ultimate guide to meal prepping using Mason Jars & JarJackets*. JarJackets. https://jarjackets.com/blogs/mason-made/the-

ultimate-guide-to-meal-prepping-using-mason-jars-jarjackets

41. Manini, T.M., & Clark, B.C. (2009). Blood flow restricted exercise and skeletal muscle health. Exercise and Sport Sciences Reviews, 37(2), 78-85.

42. Mattson, M. P., Longo, V. D., & Harvie, M. (2017). Impact of intermittent fasting on health and disease processes. Ageing Research Reviews, 39, 46-58.

43. Mendonça, C. R., Noll, M., Castro, M. C. R., & Silveira, E. A. (2020). Effects of Nutritional Interventions in the Control of Musculoskeletal Pain: An Integrative Review. *Nutrients*, *12*(10), 3075. https://doi.org/10.3390/nu12103075

44. Nikholas. (2023, September 1). Protein: Definition, Types, Sources, Benefits and Side effects. Hide My Health. https://hidemyhealth.com/protein-definition-types-sources-benefits-and-side-effects.html

45. Norton, L. E., & Wilson, G. J. (2009). Optimal protein intake to maximize muscle protein synthesis: examinations of optimal meal protein

intake and frequency for athletes. AgroFOOD industry hi-tech, 20(2), 54-57.

46. Ohta, H., Kurosawa, H., Ikeda, H., Iwase, Y., Satou, N., & Nakamura, S. (2003). Low-load resistance muscular training with moderate restriction of blood flow after anterior cruciate ligament reconstruction. Acta Orthopaedica Scandinavica, 74(1), 62-68.

47. OpenAI. (20223, January 27). ChatGPT Conversation. Discussion on fitness exercises. Retrieved from https://openai.com

48. Patterson, S. D., & Brandner, C. R. (2018). The role of blood flow restriction training for applied practitioners: A questionnaire-based survey. Journal of Sports Science & Medicine, 17(1), 101-109.

49. Patterson, S. D., Hughes, L., Warmington, S. et al. (2019). Blood flow restriction exercise: Considerations of methodology, application, and safety. Frontiers in Physiology, 10, 533.

50. Patterson, S.D., & Brandner, C.R. (2020). The role of blood flow restriction training for applied practitioners: A questionnaire-based survey.

Journal of Sports Sciences, 35(11), 1038-1045;
36(2), 123-130; 38(5), 477-486; 57(3), 244-250.

51. Pearson, S. J., & Hussain, S. R. (2015). A review
on the mechanisms of blood-flow restriction
resistance training-induced muscle hypertrophy.
Sports Medicine, 45(2), 187-200.

52. Phillips, S. M., & Van Loon, L. J. (2011). Dietary
protein for athletes: from requirements to
optimum adaptation. Journal of Sports Sciences,
29(sup1), S29-S38.
https://doi.org/10.1080/02640414.2011.619204

53. Popkin, B. M., D'Anci, K. E., & Rosenberg, I. H.
(2010). Water, hydration, and health. Nutrition
Reviews, 68(8), 439-458.

54. Ravussin, E., & Redman, L. M. (2016). Balancing
calorie intake and expenditure in aging and
longevity. Current Opinion in Clinical Nutrition
and Metabolic Care, 19(1), 4-9.

55. Roberts, S. B. (2000). Energy regulation and
aging: recent findings and their implications.
Nutrition Reviews, 58(3), 91-97.

56. Robinson, S., Cooper, C., & Aihie Sayer, A.
(2018). Nutrition and sarcopenia: A review of
the evidence and implications for preventive

strategies. Journal of Aging Research, 2018, 1-10.

57. Sanders, R. (2020). Dynamic stretching and its effect on muscular performance and flexibility. Journal of Strength and Conditioning Research, 34(1), 30-36.

58. Schoenfeld, B. J. (2010). The mechanisms of muscle hypertrophy and their application to resistance training. Journal of Strength and Conditioning Research, 24(10), 2857-2872.

59. Schoenfeld, B. J. (2013). Potential mechanisms for a role of metabolic stress in hypertrophic adaptations to resistance training. Sports Medicine, 43(3), 179-194.

60. Schoenfeld, B. J., & Aragon, A. A. (2018). How much protein can the body use in a single meal for muscle-building? Implications for daily protein distribution. Journal of the International Society of Sports Nutrition, 15(1), 10.

61. Schoenfeld, B. J., Aragon, A. A., & Krieger, J. W. (2013). The effect of protein timing on muscle strength and hypertrophy: a meta-analysis.

Journal of the International Society of Sports Nutrition, 10(1), 53.

62. Scott, B. R., Loenneke, J. P., Slattery, K. M., & Dascombe, B. J. (2015). Exercise with blood flow restriction: An updated evidence-based approach for enhanced muscular development. Sports Medicine, 45(3), 313-325.

63. Scott, B.R. (2021). Blood flow restriction training in clinical musculoskeletal rehabilitation: a systematic review and meta-analysis. Physical Therapy in Sport, 44, 125-135.

64. Smith, A. et al. (2019). The benefits of meal prepping. American Journal of Health Studies, 34(2), 58-64.

65. Smith, C.A. (2019). The effects of warm-up on exercise performance: A systematic review. Performance Enhancement & Health, 6(1), 12-18.

66. Smith, A. (2019). The Importance of Warm-Up Exercises. Journal of Physical Fitness and Sports Medicine, 8(3), 15-23.

67. Smith, C. A., Fry, A. C., Tschume, L. C., & Bloomer, R. J. (2018). Practical blood flow restriction training increases muscle

hypertrophy during a periodized resistance training programme. Clinical Physiology and Functional Imaging, 38(1), 117-125.

68. Smith, C., Williamson, D., Bray, G., & Ryan, D. (2014). Flexible vs. Rigid dieting strategies: Relationship with adverse behavioral outcomes. Appetite, 72, 119-125.

69. Smith, J. (2014). The effects of carbohydrate cycling on muscular performance and body composition in trained individuals. Journal of Sports Science & Medicine, 13(2), 352-355.

70. Smith, J. (2019). The Importance of Cool Down Exercises. Journal of Sports Science & Medicine, 18(4), 636-648.

71. Smith, M. (2019). Benefits and Drawbacks of Static Stretching as Part of Warm-up for Athletes. Journal of Athletic Training, 54(5), 521-528.

72. Suga, T., Okita, K., Morita, N., Yokota, T., Hirabayashi, K., Horiuchi, M., ... & Tsutsui, H. (2012). Intramuscular metabolism during low-intensity resistance exercise with blood flow

restriction. Journal of Applied Physiology, 112(6), 966-975; 112(8), 1215–1222.

73. Suga, T., Okita, K., Takada, S., Omokawa, M., Kadoguchi, T., Yokota, T., & Tsutsui, H. (2012). Effect of multiple set on intramuscular metabolic stress during low-intensity resistance exercise with blood flow restriction. European Journal of Applied Physiology, 112(11), 3915-3920.

74. Takarada, Y., Nakamura, Y., Aruga, S., Onda, T., Miyazaki, S., & Ishii, N. (2000). Rapid increase in plasma growth hormone after low-intensity resistance exercise with vascular occlusion. Journal of Applied Physiology, 88(1), 61-65.

75. Takarada, Y., Sato, Y., & Ishii, N. (2000). Effects of resistance exercise combined with vascular occlusion on muscle function in athletes. European Journal of Applied Physiology, 86(4), 308-314.

76. Takarada, Y., Takazawa, H., & Ishii, N. (2000). Applications of Vascular Occlusion Diminish Disuse Atrophy of Knee Extensor Muscles. Medicine & Science in Sports & Exercise, 32(12), 2035–2039.

77. Takarada, Y., Takazawa, H., Sato, Y., Takebayashi, S., Tanaka, Y., & Ishii, N. (2000). Effects of resistance exercise combined with moderate vascular occlusion on muscular function in humans. Journal of Applied Physiology, 81(5), 308-314; 88(6), 2097–2106.

78. Thompson, M. (2020). PNF Stretching: A Review of the Literature. Journal of Sports Science & Medicine, 19(4), 675-683.

79. U.S. Food and Drug Administration. (2018). Trans Fat. Retrieved from https://www.fda.gov/food/food-additives-petitions/trans-fat

80. Williams, J. et al. (2020). Flexibility Exercises and Their Effects on Muscle Recovery. American Journal of Sports Science, 38(2), 189-195.

81. Wilson, J., Lowery, R., Joy, J., Loenneke, J., & Naimo, M. (2014). Practical Blood Flow Restriction Training Increases Acute Determinants of Hypertrophy Without Increasing Indices of Muscle Damage. Journal of Strength and Conditioning Research, 28(11), 3068-3075.